PEN

TILL WE WIN

Dr Chandrakant Lahariya is a medical doctor and leading public policy and health systems expert. He has received advanced trainings in epidemiology, vaccinology, immunology and public health. He has extensive experience in disease control and elimination through his work on polio elimination, routine immunization strengthening as well as outbreak and epidemic investigations. In the last fifteen years, he has worked closely with India's leading health policymakers to develop and implement several health policies and programmes at Union and state levels. At present, his work focuses on universal health coverage, primary healthcare and health systems strengthening. In 2012, he received the Indian Council of Medical Research's (ICMR) Dr B.C. Srivastava Foundation Award for his work on translating community-based health research into public policy interventions. He is the youngest fellow ever elected to the Indian Public Health Association (IPHA).

Dr Gagandeep Kang is an infectious-disease researcher, who links community-based research to high-quality laboratory investigation. With thirty years of research at the Christian Medical College, Vellore, she has built collaborative programmes focused on enteric diseases, nutrition and the environment. She supported the development of two rotavirus vaccines made by Indian companies through clinical and laboratory testing. She serves on many advisory committees in India and internationally. She was the executive director of the Translational Health Science and Technology Institute, Faridabad, from 2016 to 2020. A fellow of many prestigious academies in India and internationally, in 2019, she became the first woman working in India to be inducted as a Fellow of the Royal Society, London.

Dr Randeep Guleria, director of the All India Institute of Medical Sciences, New Delhi, is an MD in medicine and the first DM in pulmonary medicine in the country. A world-renowned pulmonologist, he has been the chairperson and member of various policy and health forums. He has been a member of the Joint Monitoring Group of the

Government of India, created for pandemic and outbreak management in India since 2005, and has been at the forefront of the Government of India's efforts on COVID-19 pandemic preparedness and response in the country. He has published more than 350 research papers and popular articles in reputed national and international medical journals. The recipient of many awards and honours, including the Padma Shri (2015), the Dr B.C. Roy National Award in the category of Eminent Medical Person (2014), the Times Healthcare Achievers Award in the Legends category (2017), the Doctor of the Decade award by the Indian Medical Association (2017) and the National Excellence Award by the T.P. Jhunjhunwala Foundation (2017–18), Dr Guleria has delivered more than eight national orations.

TILL
WE WIN

INDIA'S FIGHT AGAINST THE
COVID-19 PANDEMIC

DR CHANDRAKANT LAHARIYA

DR GAGANDEEP KANG

DR RANDEEP GULERIA

PENGUIN BOOKS

An imprint of Penguin Random House

PENGUIN BOOKS

USA | Canada | UK | Ireland | Australia
New Zealand | India | South Africa | China

Penguin Books is part of the Penguin Random House group of companies
whose addresses can be found at global.penguinrandomhouse.com

Published by Penguin Random House India Pvt. Ltd
7th Floor, Infinity Tower C, DLF Cyber City,
Gurgaon 122 002, Haryana, India

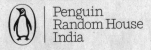

Penguin
Random House
India

First published in Penguin Books by Penguin Random House India 2020

ISBN 9780143451808

Typeset in Adobe Garamond Pro by Manipal Technologies Limited, Manipal
Printed at Thomson Press India Ltd, New Delhi

www.penguin.co.in

MIX
Paper
FSC   FSC™ C010615

This book is dedicated to the frontline healthcare workers, particularly the women from Accredited Social Health Activists (ASHAs) to nurses, who are the face of the health system

Contents

Contents

Acknowledgements

We are indebted to many people. Millions of frontline workers in health and essential services have contributed to India's fight against the COVID-19 pandemic. It is because of their courage and sustained efforts that we are able to narrate this story.

We would like to individually acknowledge our family members, friends and well-wishers.

Dr Chandrakant Lahariya

I would like to thank my parents, Urmila and Rajendra Lahariya; my wife, Anita Upadhyay Lahariya (it was much of her personal time, which I have used to write this book); and my brother Deepankar Lahariya and his wife, Rinki Gupta. Much of the first draft of this book was completed in those ten days, which I spent in the wards and corridors of the All India Institute of Medical Sciences, New Delhi (the details of that is a separate story). When this book was about to be completed, my wife and I were blessed with our daughter, Asmara. Personally speaking, this book is for her. Growing up, when she will ask about the pandemic, we will give her this book. We hope it will give her a sense of what was happening in the world when she was a foetus, safe in the womb of her mother.

Special thanks to Varun and Isha Chaudhary, Priya Karna, Sophia Lonappan, Hilde De Graeve, Rajeev Varma, Bhaskar Bhat and Payden for their contributions. I am grateful to my co-authors, Dr Gagandeep Kang and Dr Randeep Guleria, for kindly agreeing to join me in this endeavour and then being exceptionally cooperative and flexible. I have learnt many things from both of them in this journey.

Dr Gagandeep Kang

Dr Chandrakant Lahariya persuaded me that this book would be an extension of the science communication that I am passionate about, so time had to be found. My family and friends are used to my strange hours. I thank them for continuing to tolerate me and indulge my foibles.

Dr Randeep Guleria

As we go about this battle against COVID-19, I would like to take this opportunity to thank my parents for their understanding and support during these challenging times. My wife, Kiran, has been the backbone of all my efforts and nothing would have been possible without her support and patience. My son, Karandeep, daughter, Tavishi, and daughter-in-law, Niharika, deserve special thanks for always cheering me up. I am grateful to Sandeep, Raka, Neeru, Siddhartha and other members of my family for being there.

I am also thankful to Dr Chandrakant Lahariya for getting us all together and being the driving force behind this book. His efforts have made this book possible.

All three of us would like to thank the entire Penguin Random House India (PRHI) team for their excellent support and great engagement. Thank you Meru Gokhale, Shiny Das, Shantanu Ray Chaudhuri, Rachna Pratap, Gunjan Ahlawat and Peter Modoli and the entire team at PRHI.

The journey of this book began because of Premanka Goswami, who impressed upon us the importance of writing it. He helped us sail through this, navigating difficult timelines. Thanks, Premanka.

It is not possible to name all those who made direct or indirect contributions but thanks indeed to each one of you, who are not mentioned here because of space constraints. You know you have contributed to shape this book and bend the curve of the pandemic downwards.

Preface

When India's cities—such as Gwalior, Vellore or Delhi (or Bengaluru and Mumbai, for that matter)—receive an hour-long pre-monsoon or monsoon shower, the evening news or newspapers carry almost identical headlines and images of those cities. Predominantly, images of waterlogging and stranded citizens take over the news cycle. Based on such reports, someone staying in a different city may get the impression that the deluge affected the entire city. It creates a negative image about the place being unliveable. In many of these reports, old images are flashed to make the point that little has changed for years or decades. Almost always, the local government and administration are blamed and termed ineffective. While the reports and visuals might be true, in a majority of cases, the problem might be localized and other areas in the city would have faced no issue, which might be because the same administration or agency made efforts that were successful in preventing the problem. So, to present a balanced view, while highlighting civic and other issues is important, it is also equally critical to bring to light the efforts that were efficient and successful.

The COVID-19 pandemic is an unprecedented health challenge for all of humanity. Even countries with excellent infrastructure have been severely affected. As the pandemic accelerated, there were apprehensions that with a population of nearly 1.38 billion, it would be a nightmare for India. In the fourth week of March 2020, an international group made projections that India would have hundreds of millions of infections and lakhs of deaths, a prospect that was terrifying for everyone.

India's first case of coronavirus was reported on 30 January 2020. In February–early March 2020, the pandemic was unfolding in many countries, especially in Europe. Hospitals were overburdened; there was need for additional ventilators; people were being refused admission to hospitals and there was a relatively high death rate due to COVID-19.

The challenges in healthcare infrastructure and services in India are widely known and noted across various circles. Further, given the lack of a robust laboratory surveillance system, the testing capacity for a new virus was very limited. In addition, India had zero production capacity for many items essential for healthcare, including personal protective equipment (PPE) coverall, which are indispensable for the safety of health staff involved in contact tracing, inpatient care and testing. Hospital and ICU beds, ventilators and other essential equipment were limited.

The implementation of social distancing and basic hygiene, which required wider participation of communities, was a practical challenge. Population density and overcrowded workplaces, dwellings and transport added to the operational challenges. Further, since health is a state subject in the Indian Constitution policies may be suggested by the Centre but the responsibility to implement lies with the state governments. Therefore there were apprehensions about the preparedness of states and their ability to respond to the pandemic.

Over the past nine months in India, policymakers, health experts, hospital staff, community-level workers, entire administration and communities have jointly and separately fought the pandemic. There have been stumbles, but we have found a way to get up and start walking again.

Every day has offered something new. Policies have evolved with the situation, and we have frequently found that the information one had before going to bed proved to be redundant on waking up. Tracking the pandemic required extensive reading, sifting through information through a filter of reliability, of follow-ups with colleagues and experts around the world to get updates on what had changed since the last update. With a new pathogen, experts needed to build on existing knowledge and rapidly emerging information to develop new guidelines in the initial stages, and to keep updating those guidelines with new information from different parts of the world.

The pandemic has had social and economic challenges, in addition to the impact on health. While the lockdown resulted in slowing down transmission, it caused a lot of problems to the migrants and poor across the country. In the initial stages of the pandemic, the fear of spread of infection and the stigma associated with the disease resulted in health workers being attacked while they were involved in contact tracing. Hospital staff and COVID-19 positive patients were stigmatized and discriminated against in their workplaces and where they lived. People in need of essential health services other than for COVID-19, such as pregnant women and those with cancer, diabetes and hypertension, faced challenges in accessing these. These stories were splattered across newspapers and television channels. Alongside, people working in response to COVID-19 were termed 'corona warriors' and their role began to be highlighted in the media, and even in advertising, such as on packaging for yoghurt and other foods.

This has been an unprecedented time for the health sector and particularly for those dealing with infectious diseases. Newspapers and television channels are full of news about COVID-19, the spread of the pandemic and the availability or lack of hospital services. There is almost no one whose life has not been touched by the pandemic and for the first time, challenges related to infections and health issues have become subjects of household discussions. Words such as quarantine, isolation, epidemiology, public health, immunity and sero-survey have become familiar to journalists and vast swathes of society. People from all walks of life seem to be discussing PPE, ventilators, plasma therapy, hydroxychloroquine, hospital beds, oxygen beds and other aspects which until a few months ago were not part of popular discourse. Everyone is now asking when a vaccine against COVID-19 will be available and every single news item on new treatments is explained and discussed in the media.

In the past nine months, elected leaders, politicians and policymakers have deliberated on the health-sector challenges in the country like never before. They have consulted nationally and globally with experts to formulate and deliver policies related to testing, quarantine and treatment and are now debating further on vaccines and the opportunities these may afford for recovery.

Policymakers, health experts and citizens alike are sensitized about the challenges faced by the health system in India. We also recognize that improvements in health and well-being require action at all levels, from individuals for healthy behaviours, to experts for synthesis of scientific information to provide advice, to the policymaker for short- and long-term changes. While fighting this pandemic is the urgent need of today, this is an opportunity for all key stakeholders (policymakers, experts and the public) to strengthen overall health services so that we are better prepared for what is needed every day and, in particular, for the next pandemic.

The first approaches to controlling the pandemic are 'Test, Trace, Treat and Isolate': basic fundamentals for any emergent infectious disease and yet the most critical pillars to deal with the crisis, until solutions like drugs and vaccines can be developed. These are also linked to the fields of microbiology, public health and epidemiology, and clinical medicine, among others.

Each of one of us specializes in one or more of these areas. We have been involved in the pandemic response in our individual and professional capacities. We have had experience in past outbreaks and epidemics in India. With a long-term association with India's health sector and an insider perspective on how the country has responded to the pandemic, we aim to offer a long-term overview of what is needed to improve the system.

We believe that an informed public is the key stakeholder in pandemic response. For any infectious disease, the behaviour and actions of people from every part of society are an integral part of achieving success in disease control. Evolving a 'new normal', managing future spread and boosting the ability of health services to provide care when and where needed are dependent on the equal participation of people. This book delves into those aspects as well, addressing how people can adopt a healthier lifestyle. This approach to prevention of infection was always useful, but has become even more relevant now.

The impact of health on society is now centre stage. The impact on the economy is obvious, even if its full extent will be clear only with time. The government has announced a series of financial stimulus packages, the value and implementation of which has been widely debated. The Fifteenth Finance Commission has revisited the health recommendations in the wake of the pandemic.

A remarkable aspect of the pandemic has been how much it affected every aspect of society. In addition, with the mushrooming of 'experts' on viruses, epidemiology, mathematical modelling, clinical research, logistics and economy, we had an explosion of information and advice to people, from the duration and location of quarantine to potential prevention, immunity boosting, treatments and vaccine development.

As our understanding of the virus and its spread increased, we went from early expert advice that limited masks to healthcare settings to masks becoming part of our everyday attire. Hand sanitizers and handwashing have almost become an emblem of responsibility. 'Social (or physical) distancing', working from home and virtual meetings became the norm within a few months. People repeat complex names such as tocilizumab, remdesivir and hydroxychloroquine as if they have been familiar with these terms for years. Those who would rarely consider vaccination are enquiring about the availability of COVID-19 vaccines. The world has completely changed.

The change is being termed the 'new normal'. How do we live with the virus and still function as individuals, families, students, teachers and professionals? What do we need to do to protect ourselves and others? What are the guarantees afforded and assurance provided by our behaviours? What are the risks and benefits of our actions?

Nine months into the pandemic, we are still at an early stage of the human experience with SARS-Coronavirus 2, but given the widespread misinformation (termed 'infodemic') and lack of easily understandable information on critical aspects of the virus, the disease and control measures, we believe that this book will be useful for every citizen. Whether students, homemakers, office goers, an IT professional or a culinary expert, a policewoman or a bureaucrat, we argue that we need everyone in India to pitch in in the war against COVID-19.

The pandemic is a long way from being over. Everyone needs to protect her/himself, family members and community and society as a whole, as best as they can. While no perfect protection is possible till the pandemic is over in all parts of the world, the risk of infection can be greatly reduced if we all follow a few approaches and strategies and a few simple health recommendations, which we share in this book.

This book narrates the story of India's fight against the pandemic. It is an evolving story, but with enough to provide key information which each citizen needs or would like to know about how the pandemic emerged and grew, what was done, what continues to be done and what the future may hold for all of us.

All three of us were trained as medical doctors and then received our training in specialized fields. Since then, we have worked with patients, and in communities and laboratories. While we have published extensively in academic medical journals, written chapters for medical textbooks, taught graduate and postgraduate medical students, delivered public lectures and seminars, writing a book for general readers was not foremost on our minds.

But the pandemic changed everything around us; it changed the way all of us lived. We have had a pandemic before, just a decade ago with swine flu or H1N1, but it was much less severe in terms of spread and mortality rates. Health systems were never tested as they have been in 2020.

This book has many threes. There are three authors. The core strategy in the initial pandemic response involved three steps: test, trace and treat. The core technologies that need to be developed for managing the pandemic are three: diagnostic tests, drugs and vaccines. We also had three major reasons for writing this book.

One, the response to COVID-19 is multi-sectoral. Without the engagement of experts from multiple fields within medicine, biomedical sciences and public health, we could not have evolved a strategy for detection, management or control. The 'test, trace and treat' strategy for effective response to the pandemic requires expertise and understanding of microbiology, public health and curative medicine, respectively. Amongst the three authors, we have specialized in different areas and believe that our collective perspective builds a comprehensive picture of the pandemic so far, India's response and what the uncertain future may hold. As a disclaimer, however, the perspectives and views in this book do not reflect the official work of the institutions and organizations we are affiliated with. All views and perspectives in this book are personal and should be attributed to the authors alone.

Second, we have dealt with many people and policymakers during this period. Many of these interactions revealed that despite the constant news cycle, there continue to be gaps in perception and much misinformation and misconception about the response to the pandemic. We want to build on that increased interest in health systems as well as in clinical medicine to explore how best this opportunity can be utilized for better health and better epidemic and pandemic preparedness in India. Once the pandemic is over, every one of us who has lived through this would be keen to get an overview of how India fought the pandemic. We should ask ourselves what we have learnt. This book could be a guide for such reflections. Additionally, in the future, young people may be interested in a record of India's response to the pandemic.

Third, although the story is incomplete, we want to provide a sense of the challenges faced in the initial days of the pandemic, with a focus on India, and also narrate the story of how we are gearing up for a 'new normal'. We have worked with many people and policymakers during this period as well as in the past. What was a revelation to us was that there was no single, common understanding of the different aspects of health and health systems. But there is an interest in understanding the challenges and solutions. We as authors wanted to build on that increased interest to explore how best this opportunity can be utilized for a healthy India.

Hope you would enjoy reading the book and write to us with your suggestions, feedback and comments.

October 2020   Dr Chandrakant Lahariya
                                              Dr Gagandeep Kang
                                              Dr Randeep Guleria

Introduction

The novel Coronavirus (known initially as 2019-nCoV, later renamed SARS-CoV-2 or Severe Acute Respiratory Syndrome Coronavirus-2) emerged in late 2019 and early 2020. The first human case was officially reported from Wuhan in Hubei province of China on 31 December 2019. In India, the first case was reported from Kerala on 30 January 2020. By February 2020, it became clear that this was on a scale not witnessed for many decades and arguably since the Spanish Flu of 1918–19. It was declared a pandemic by the World Health Organization (WHO) on 11 March 2020.

In India, concerns escalated even though for the first month after the initial infections in Kerala, no cases were detected. The worries were justified. India does not have as effective and efficient a health system as, say, Japan or South Korea or other nations in the West. The challenges are wide-ranging: from the shortage of health facilities and doctors, nurses and hospital beds to the quality of care and the complexity of a healthcare system that has not just private and public health providers but also multiple systems of medicine, from Ayurveda to homeopathy, and a diverse group of actors, such as the 'Bangali' doctors and other unqualified providers in rural and poor urban areas. Moreover, India's urban population density and poor living and working conditions make it ideal for the virus to spread across vast swathes of the country rapidly.

On 24 March 2020, a modelling-based study led by reputed international institutes projected that if there were no interventions, India could have 30 to 40 crore (300 to 400 million) cases of COVID-19 by July 2020. Though the majority of cases were projected to be mild, with such high numbers of infections, the study estimated a peak hospitalization of around 10 to 20 lakh (one to two million) and the need for nearly one million ventilators. Even as the report came out, India went into a lockdown.

However, against the grim projections, India has reported COVID-19 cases and deaths far below every 'disease modelling' estimate made in the earlier stages of the pandemic. It is partly indicative of the success of the many interventions undertaken, but there's no denying the upheavals we have faced. Given that the whole world, including the most developed nations, has been severely affected, perhaps much—if not everything—of what we have faced was unavoidable. Understanding what made a difference and what else we could have done is important today, and for the future. The response to a pandemic is expected to have hits and misses. While each hit or success needs to be celebrated and credited, the misses should be used for learning. In fact, our biggest failure would be not learning from this experience.

It will require distance and time to narrate the story of the virus and its consequences with any degree of objectivity. Meanwhile, this book seeks to document and celebrate the efforts of those who have contributed to India's response to the pandemic so far, and to share some ideas on what needs to be done to prepare for the next epidemic and pandemic by strengthening health systems in India.

The book is organized in four sections and eleven chapters.

The first section, 'Understanding the Challenge', discusses that pathogens (or disease-causing agents) are a part of life. Pathogens cause diseases which may be limited to a single site, such as the urinary bladder or the liver, while others, called systemic diseases, such as many fevers, may affect more than one organ. If it is a respiratory virus, the pathogen and the human host could combine to create a challenge that is unpredictable in timing and scale, resulting in pandemics. There are two chapters in this section. Chapter 1 gives an overview of viruses, their long association with human beings and how they influence co-evolution. Chapter 2 provides an introduction to coronaviruses, of which SARS-CoV-2 is the most recent in humans after the Middle East Respiratory Syndrome coronavirus (MERS CoV). It discusses how this new virus is a bigger challenge than all previous coronaviruses. The chapter also provides a brief history of viral pandemics.

The second section, 'Mounting a Response', comprising four chapters, brings to light how India continues to respond to COVID-19. Chapter 3 focuses on the period from early January 2020 to 24 March 2020. Chapter 4 captures the actions and activities from 25 March 2020 to 31 May 2020, when India went through four phases of lockdown. This period intended to improve healthcare systems including laboratory services and develop epidemiological understanding to halt the spread of the virus. There were many focal outbreaks in a number of Indian states, which provided learnings and lessons. Chapter 5 focuses on the period starting 1 June 2020, with Unlock 1. It was hoped that things would open up and life would return to normal. However, soon after opening up, it was realized that while the spread had slowed down, all states were not adequately prepared to handle the situation. Cases surged in many parts of the country and specially in the cities and states of Delhi, Bengaluru, Chennai, Hyderabad, Pune and Kerala. The disease began spreading to smaller cities and districts, reaching the remotest corners. A few months into the pandemic and it became increasingly clear that an effective response to the disease required rigorous public health measures (to reduce the cases and spread), a robust laboratory network (for early identification of cases) and sufficient hospital bed capacity (to treat patients). Chapter 6 narrates the stories of frontline workers who fought against all odds to ensure that the disease does not spread. Doctors and nurses died in the line of duty, as did police personnel, sanitation workers, ward boys and frontline health staff. We also look at community participation and engagement, the interventions of panchayats and the Resident Welfare Associations (RWAs) in responding to the pandemic.

The third section, Science, Solidarity and Hope, has two chapters which focus on vaccines and therapies, the interventions of science in addressing the virus. Probably for the first time in history, medical research and vaccine development are happening in the public eye and are being reported in real time. If public health (and epidemiology) and medical care have been at the core of the response so far, in the period ahead, science and research, including vaccines and therapies, will determine the course of the pandemic.

The fourth section, 'Getting Future-Ready', delves into what is needed going ahead to respond to the pandemic effectively. This section has three chapters, one each on proposed suggestions for a sustained and effective response to the pandemic, broader policy suggestions on how to strengthen overall Indian health systems, and how to stay safe and healthy at individual and community levels in the new normal.

Chapter 9 details and proposes a few immediate policy and operational interventions for authorities at every level. Chapter 10 builds on the understanding that health challenges in India have come to the forefront like never before. Every stakeholder has become aware of these challenges. Elected leaders and other policymakers are keen to act and intervene to improve the health system. The opportunity created by this pandemic and the learnings, if used effectively, can pave the way for better health for every citizen. In Chapter 11 we provide practical tips to the readers on how to stay safe and healthy. These tips have been addressed to individuals, families, communities as well as specific common settings such as offices, during travel, in flights, etc.

Many of the chapters in the book have a section titled Frequently Asked Questions (FAQs) which deals with the questions around the pandemic we have been often asked over the last few months.

The book ends with an afterword.

This is not an exhaustive documentation of India's response to the pandemic. What we provide is an overview. In spite of many challenges, we emphasize that India's response to the pandemic has already resulted in many positive developments.

Individuals and communities have, on their own, stepped up efforts to prevent disease spread, often in the face of little or incomplete information. More people are following and adhering to the non-pharmacological interventions of masks or face covers, handwashing and physical distancing. These three continue to be amongst the most powerful tools to stop the pandemic. The COVID-19 testing capacity has increased, with a network of around 2000 laboratories—in public and private sector combined—conducting more than a million COVID-19 tests every day.

Millions of frontline workers have demonstrated that contact tracing can be done in India, and with very high fidelity. They have visited millions of households across India to trace and follow up on the contacts of COVID-19 positive cases as well as for clinical surveillance. Mobile based applications, such as 'Arogya Setu', and other state-specific applications were effectively used for contact tracing and to deliver public health messages.

India has created an overall capacity of nearly 1.7 million COVID-19 beds across all states, by repurposing existing facilities or adding new beds. In addition, home isolation of mild cases is slowly becoming a proven and effective strategy, which also underscores the role of community and people's participation in the collective response and management.

India has stepped up research and development for COVID-19 vaccines, drugs and other therapies. By mid-October 2020, nearly thirty indigenous candidate vaccines and many therapies were under pre-clinical and clinical stages of trials. A few vaccines are in phase II/III of clinical trials. Given its large vaccine manufacturing capacity, India is expected to be a major contributor to the global supply of COVID-19 vaccines.

Many innovations have been put into practice to ensure the availability of health services. These include providing legal status to teleconsultation for medical care, legalizing home delivery of medicines and the engagement of AYUSH providers for preventive and promotive health services. A number of regulatory measures, such as capping the price of laboratory tests and charges for hospital beds in the private sector, have been initiated to ensure access to care. There were other developments at high policy levels, including, for the first time, the final report of the Fifteenth Finance Commission having a dedicated chapter on health.

This is thus a story of people's participation, perseverance and positivity in achieving a common goal. The real success of these efforts would entail putting these lessons and learnings in the service of a much-improved health system for every Indian citizen. A system built on the foundation of a stronger primary healthcare system, with sufficient provision of preventive, promotive and other public health services.

We also urge you, the reader, to use this information to consider how you can make that happen, for yourself, for those in your family and your neighbourhood. It could be by adopting healthier lifestyles, sharing knowledge with others, as well as by strengthening systems by holding local service providers and elected leaders accountable. There are so many

ways you can use the information in this book and we leave
that to your discretion and judgement.

As the world watched, one of the world's most populous
slums, Dharavi, in Mumbai, was identified as a potentially
unstoppable hotspot for COVID-19. However, the
experience from this densely populated slum showed that
determined and coordinated action can fight against any
formidable challenge. If this virus can be handled, many
other annual challenges of dengue, chikungunya and other
infections should also be planned for and countered. If we
can trace many contacts for COVID-19 cases, can't we adopt
a similar approach of trace and treat for tuberculosis (TB)
cases in India? That can help in accelerating the target of TB
elimination from India and achieve 'TB Mukt Bharat'. Can
people's participation in preventive and promotive health
interventions be leveraged to revert the 'silent epidemic' of
diabetes and hypertension in India? The answer to these and
many other questions is, yes.

The COVID-19 pandemic has, in a way, brought society
together against a common threat, which requires the close
collaboration of various sectors and contribution of health
staff and every member of society. Such coordination,
collaboration and partnership need to continue beyond the
pandemic to make India a nation with robust health systems
and healthy people.

Section I

Understanding the Challenge

1

Viruses, Ecosystems and the Inevitability of Pandemics

How many humans are estimated to be on the Earth?
8,000,000,000

How many viruses are estimated to be on the planet?
10,000,000,000,000,000,000,000,000,000,000

For every human being, how many viruses are there on this planet?
~125,000,000,000,000,000,000,000

Do humans represent the peak of evolution or viruses? As humans have evolved, they have become more and more complex, in their biology and in their functioning, while viruses have become simpler and simpler—getting rid of genes they do not need, to the point where viruses hijack the host cells they infect and use their machinery to replicate.

For all the complexity of life, every living organism is made mainly from about thirty molecules of some of the most abundant elements in the universe. It seems incredible that the first living organisms came into being just a few hundred million years after the formation of the Earth. The first microbes appeared approximately 4 billion years ago. Compare that to our hominid ancestors who appeared only about 18 million years ago and *Homo sapiens*, the species to which we belong, who evolved only about 300,000 years ago.

In studying the evolution of different forms of life, tracing viruses is difficult because they do not leave fossils. Viruses infect every living organism, from bacteria to elephants, tomatoes to starfish. Scientists try to piece together histories of viruses by tracking their genes. Viruses make copies of themselves in infected cells and sometimes leave their genes behind, at times by stitching their genes into the genes of their host.

We do not know exactly how viruses evolved. A number of possible ways have been proposed, but none explains all that we know about viruses: they could have come from free living cells that became simpler, they could have come from pieces of DNA (deoxyribonucleic acid) and RNA (ribonucleic acid) that escaped from host cells and acquired a protein coat, or they could have co-evolved with their hosts. In the past decade, an interesting way of studying virus evolution has emerged that has moved away from studying genes to viral proteins. By looking at the folding of proteins from cells and viruses, Gustavo Caetano-Anolles, from the University of Illinois, found that viruses have sixty-six unique protein folds that seem to have appeared about 1.5 billion years ago.

Despite the limited number and commonality of proteins, viruses are not all the same. Human immunodeficiency virus or HIV, which is a virus we recognized only in the 1980s, is thought to have actually emerged in humans in the 1930s. The HIV belongs to an interesting family—the retroviruses. Although HIV is relatively new to humans, retroviruses are not. Retroviruses reverse the normal flow of information inside a cell, which is usually from the DNA to the RNA, with an enzyme called reverse transcriptase that instead copies information from the RNA to the DNA. These DNA signatures from retroviruses which are inserted into the genome of the host cell, and can be left behind to be inherited by the next generation, are called endogenous retroviruses. In fact, in humans 1 to 5 per cent of the genome is made up of these viral signatures, which have been left over from the infection of our distant ancestors and may have influenced our evolution to what we are today.

There are all kinds of odd viruses. A few years ago, French scientists were trying to classify an organism that looked like a bacterium but had a very different genome. This mystery microbe, which had more than a thousand genes, was actually a giant virus. It was named the mimivirus for 'mimicking microbe', and, subsequently, many more of these physically and genetically large viruses have been found. Several viruses that are very large seem to infect simple organisms such as amoebae and algae, indicating that these may be more ancient than smaller viruses which infect more complex organisms.

Despite all of the common features of viruses and their ability to copy and spread their genomes, viruses still remain a mystery. It is estimated that there are almost 100 million different types of viruses and that at any time there are 10^{31} viruses on the planet, making them the most numerous microbes on the Earth, with their numbers being about ten times more than that of bacteria. And they are ubiquitous; there are 10 billion viruses per litre of sea water, they float in the air, and their signatures are found in almost every living cell.

Although viruses are everywhere, we did not know about them, or even speculate about their distinctive characteristics, until the nineteenth century. Edward Jenner developed the first vaccine, using the cowpox virus to protect against the disfiguring, deadly disease of smallpox, without knowing anything about viruses and their life cycle. Similarly, Louis Pasteur used the principle of weakening an infectious agent by growing it outside its original host to produce the first rabies vaccine. But it was not until 1892 that Dmitri Ivanovsky showed that filtering the sap from diseased tobacco plants with a filter that retained the bacteria still allowed other tobacco plants on which the filtered sap was placed to become infected. This revealed that there were infectious agents smaller than bacteria. Martinus Beijerinck, a Dutch botanist and microbiologist, from his experiments on tobacco disease, inferred that this was due to an infectious fluid containing a 'soluble filterable agent' that was not bacteria. He named them viruses, derived from 'poison, sap, slimy fluid'.

While bacteria could be seen under the microscope, seeing viruses was not possible until the early twentieth century, so scientists tried to understand what these 'filterable agents' or viruses were capable of, with very interesting experiments. Frederick Twort, an English scientist, tried to grow viruses, thinking that the smallpox vaccine grown in the skin of calves may need an 'essential substance' that was made by bacteria which could be frequently found in the vaccine. In 1914, he discovered that when he grew the bacteria, in some areas, the bacteria just would not grow, and taking material from that area killed other bacteria as well. Similar work was also done by Félix d'Hérelle a self-taught French-Canadian scientist, who showed that bacteria could be killed by a transmissible filterable substance, resulting in the 'Twort-d'Hérelle phenomenon'. Although it was not recognized at the time, even earlier, in 1896, Ernest Hankin, an English bacteriologist had described a unique phenomenon, that the waters of the Ganga river could destroy *Vibrio cholerae*, the bacteria that cause cholera. He showed that the effect persisted even if the water was filtered, but was destroyed by heating the water.

We now know that these effects are caused by bacteriophages, viruses that destroy bacteria. The most typical picture of a bacteriophage is of a tiny machine-like structure, which attaches to bacteria and injects its DNA into the bacterial cell, causing it to make more phages and self-destruct or wait until the time is right to make many more daughter phages that can then infect other cells.

This ability of phages is now being used to destroy bacteria that can cause life-threatening infections. In 2015, Tom Patterson, a scientist who was on vacation in Egypt, developed acute pancreatitis followed by an infection with a dangerous bacterium called *Acinetobacter baumannii*, on which no antibiotic had any effect. As Tom got sicker, his wife, Steffanie Strathdee, also a scientist, arranged for him to brought back to the United States of America and started to look for potential cures. Phage therapy, which involves the search for phages that can destroy specific bacteria, has been used for decades in Russia and several eastern European countries, where access to high-end antibiotics has been limited. Steffanie persuaded a scientist in Texas and the US Navy to find phages for Tom's strain of *Acinetobacter*. As told in *The Perfect Predator: A Scientist's Race to Save Her Husband from a Deadly Superbug*, they were ultimately successful.

Beyond treatment of human disease, bacteriophages and other viruses interact with all forms of life to maintain a balance. Viruses need a host cell to be able to replicate. Thus the question arises, whether viruses are truly living organisms, since they cannot survive on their own. The question often asked is—*are viruses alive*? In a formal sense, viruses are not alive, if we define life by the seven processes: movement, respiration, sensitivity, nutrition, excretion, reproduction and growth. However, viruses have genetic information, a characteristic shared by every other living thing, and they reproduce, which in their interactions with host cells completes their 'life' or reproductive cycle.

Viruses remained a mystery because they had not been seen, and experiments to determine their composition developed slowly in the first few decades of the twentieth century. Although the electron microscope was developed in the 1930s, the first images of viruses came from X-rays of crystallized virus by Wendell Stanley in 1935. Stanley also showed that viruses consisted of protein and nucleic acids. In 1941, the tobacco mosaic virus was shown to be a skinny stick-like shape by electron microscopy. The images dispelled any doubt of their existence. Viruses consisted of genetic material in a coat of protein molecules.

Although many of the early experiments were done with viruses of bacteria and plants, particularly tobacco, an economically important crop, the identification of viruses as agents of human disease was not far behind. It had been proposed by Carlos Finlay, a Cuban physician, that yellow fever was transmitted by mosquitoes. This theory was shown to be correct through experiments on humans by Walter Reed, and led to the destruction of mosquito habitats in the Panama by William Gorgas, and the subsequent building of the Panama Canal, which opened in 1914. The yellow fever virus was isolated by Max Theiler, who made many contributions to virology, including the development of a yellow fever vaccine.

While being able to identify the structure of viruses and show that they were made of proteins and nucleic acids was important, further major advances happened when methods to grow viruses outside whole plants and animals (and humans) were developed. In 1913, the cowpox or vaccinia virus was grown in fragments of guinea pig corneal tissue, and then in hens' kidneys, but tissue culture, or the growing of cells outside the host, was standardized and adopted in the 1950s, a major advance that led to the production of the first poliovirus vaccines.

Despite the advances being made in virology through the first half of the twentieth century, the influenza pandemic of 1918–19 was attributed to a bacterium, *Haemophilus influenzae*. It was not until 1931, when the virus was grown in fertilized chicken eggs, that it was recognized that the causative agent was not a bacterium.

The associations between viruses and diseases increased over the next few decades, and new tools were used to identify, characterize and manipulate viruses. The differences between viruses with a DNA genome and those with RNA, that is, the presence of genes on separate strands instead of being linked up together, all influenced how viruses adapted and evolved. Viruses were shown to cause some forms of cancer. This understanding of the association led to treatments and vaccines for cure or prevention of different forms of disease.

Since the early twentieth century, our knowledge of viruses has grown enormously. We have developed vaccines and drugs to treat viral infections. We use viruses as tools for carrying genes into cells for gene therapy, we use them to make vaccines, treat superbug infections and we even use them to target and kill cancer cells.

But despite all that we know and can do, there are times when viruses can change the world and we need to scramble to keep up. The year 2020 is an example.

What Is a Pandemic?

The word 'pandemic' is not related to severity of the disease. It indicates the geographical area and the extent of population spread. There are three terms used in public health to describe situations depending on the extent of spread: outbreaks, epidemics and pandemics.

An 'outbreak' is a sudden rise in cases of a disease in a small geographical area within a defined political boundary. Outbreaks can be as small as three or four linked cases, for example, a food-related illness, or as large as several thousand people.

An 'epidemic' is the rapid spread of disease among a larger number of people in a vast geographical area within a short time. For some diseases, specific rates are defined. For example, in 1996, the UK defined an influenza epidemic as a time when the rate of consultations for flu-like symptoms in a sample of reporting by general practitioners exceeds 400 per 100,000 people in one week.

A 'pandemic' refers to the worldwide spread of disease. The US Centers for Disease Control and Prevention defines a pandemic as 'an epidemic that has spread over several countries or continents, usually affecting a large number of people'.

As opposed to sudden increases, labelled as outbreaks, epidemics and pandemics, there are endemic diseases, which are present all the time in the population. All these different terms derive from Latin words ('demos' from people, 'epi'-upon, 'pan'-all, 'en'-in).

Since this classification of disease is based on geographical spread, a disease that initially starts as an outbreak can move towards being an epidemic and finally to the stage of a pandemic. COVID-19 was an outbreak in Wuhan, which became an epidemic when it spread to other areas in Asia and then moved rapidly towards being declared a pandemic.

If the disease persists around the world, it is possible that it will become an endemic disease. Other examples are rotavirus infections, which cause acute watery diarrhoea in children, and seasonal coronavirus infections that cause common colds among people of practically all ages and in all geographies.

There has been a fair amount of confusion about the difference between outbreaks, epidemics and pandemics and the definitions used by public health agencies. The WHO, while revising the International Health Regulations (IHR) in 2005, developed a classification of what are called public health emergencies of international concern (PHEIC).

Epidemics and Pandemics through History

About 5000 years ago, an epidemic struck in north-eastern China in an archaeological site called Hamin Mangha and wiped out an entire population. Dead bodies of children, and young and old people were found stuffed inside a house that had been burnt down. The epidemic spread so quickly that there was no time for proper burials. The village was abandoned and never inhabited again.

The first documented smallpox outbreak dates back to 1350 BCE. The virus killed nearly 30 per cent of those infected, scarring and blinding many of the survivors. The scourge persisted through history, until a vaccine was finally made in 1798, but the uptake was incomplete. In the twentieth century alone, 300 million people died of smallpox. Fortunately, through targeted use of the vaccine and dedicated efforts of a range of partners, the last human case due to natural infection was reported in 1977 and the disease was declared eradicated in 1980.

The Plague of Athens in ancient Greece in 430–427 BCE killed 100,000 people during a war, with an agent that may have been Ebola or typhoid. The Antonine Plague around 165–180 CE was probably brought into the Roman Empire by soldiers returning home after a war against Parthia. The Plague of Cyprian in 250–271 CE in the Mediterranean is estimated to have killed 5000 people in a day in Rome alone. It is not known what caused the epidemic, but the description is dramatic: 'The bowels, relaxed into a constant flux, discharge the bodily strength [and] a fire originated in the marrow ferments into wounds of the fauces (an area of the mouth)'.[1] Cyprian described the epidemic as signalling the end of the world. In 2014, archaeologists in Luxor found a mass burial site of plague victims, with bodies covered with a thick layer of lime, which was used as a disinfectant as well as evidence of a bonfire used to burn plague victims.

There have been many, many epidemics, both recorded and unrecorded. In the fourteenth century, the Black Death travelled from Asia to Europe, wiping out populations wherever it spread. The plague bacillus, *Yersinia pestis*, spread by fleas on infected rodents. About half of the population of Europe died. Bodies were thrown on the streets and buried in mass graves. This changed the course of history; with no manpower, the world had to adapt to a new way of functioning, leading to better working conditions, as it was seen that those who survived were better nourished.

The Black Death persisted across Europe for centuries with the last major outbreak in Great Britain. The plague began in April 1665 and caused an exodus from London led by King Charles II. It spread rapidly through the hot summer months, killing about 100,000 people. About 15 per cent of the population of London died.

There are also diseases that, by their mode of spread, have caused repeated pandemics. Two well-known examples are

---

[1] Available at https://www.livescience.com/46335-remains-of-ancient-egypt-epidemic-found.html.

cholera and influenza. In the past 200 years there have been seven cholera pandemics. The first erupted in India in 1817 and over seven years affected many countries, killing many British soldiers whose graves are found all over India, and almost 10,000 people in Java, Indonesia. The second cholera pandemic which started a decade later, reached Russia, Europe and the US. The quarantine measures imposed on the populations of these countries resulted in riots that were called the 'Cholera Riots' and had to be quelled with force. The third pandemic started in 1846, and was remarkable in the scale of deaths with a million people dying in Russia alone. James Polk, the US President, died of cholera after a trip to Louisiana and was buried in an infectious disease grave, as required by local law. The third pandemic was also notable in history because it was during this pandemic that John Snow laid the foundations of infectious disease epidemiology, by tracing the potential source of a cholera outbreak in London to a pump in Broad Street. Three more pandemics followed, but in the sixth pandemic, which started in 1961, it was found that rehydration was the key to surviving cholera, and intravenous and later oral rehydration solutions began to be used. Although the availability and use of rehydration is not as much as it should be, this single approach is believed to have saved billions of lives.

In the early 1990s, a new strain of *V. cholerae* emerged. This was the O139 strain that originated, like most cholera pandemics do, in the Bay of Bengal. Over a few years, O139 spread around the world, almost replacing the strain that had been there before, and then its numbers began to decrease and the older strains came back. The interplay between strains, environmental conditions and disease outbreaks is a fascinating area of exploration, and every year we learn more and more. Cholera is an ancient disease, and we now know how to treat patients, we have vaccines, we understand a lot about spread, but we have still not be able to control its spread or eliminate it. A seeding of cholera from Asia to Haiti in 2010 led to a raging, prolonged outbreak that only came under control when vaccines were used. Even now, an estimated 1.5 to 3 million cholera cases and around 150,000 deaths are reported annually, and this is likely to be a conservative estimate because we do not have systematic ways of testing and reporting.

The Great Influenza Pandemic of 1918–19

In the context of the current pandemic, a lot of references and comparisons are made to the influenza pandemic of 1918–19. Although the cause of the illness was not identified correctly at the time, we know now that it was a strain of the H1N1 influenza virus, which had genes that came from bird influenza viruses. Even though it was labelled the Spanish Flu, because the Spanish press was the first and consistent reporter of the illness, while other countries suppressed the news, we actually do not know where the virus originated. We do know that it spread across the world during 1918–19 and about one-third of the world's population was infected, and an estimated 40 to 50 million people died.

The disease was seen in some parts of the world with more than one peak; there was an early smaller peak in cases followed by a second very high peak a few months later. In smaller communities, the virus came in and wiped out almost the entire population. Unusually, it killed young healthy people between twenty and forty years of age, as well as the very young and the old.

We still have little understanding of all of the factors that made the virus so devastating, even though in the early 2000s, through an incredible series of investigations, the virus sequence was recovered from the body of an Inuit woman who had been buried in the permafrost. The virus was synthesized and studied, and it was shown that the virus induced a severe reaction or cytokine storm in infected animals, perhaps explaining why younger people died.

During the 1918 epidemic, the tools that could be used for control were limited. There were no vaccines and no antibiotics (and antivirals). Much as we are doing today, masks and disinfection were recommended, good personal hygiene was emphasized. Isolation and quarantine were implemented when possible. Limitations were imposed on public gatherings by local authorities. But the virus swept through the populations, overwhelming healthcare systems and killing one in ten of those who were infected.

In India, the influenza pandemic is believed to have started with the return of soldiers from the Great War or the First World War to Bombay (now Mumbai) in June 1918. The disease was thus referred to as Bombay Fever or Bombay Influenza. The outbreak moved from western India to the east and north within months. There were three waves, with the second causing the greatest mortality as had happened in other parts of the world. Similar to age patterns elsewhere, younger people were severely affected, but in India, women suffered disproportionately. The severity and high mortality might have been driven by malnutrition due to a failed monsoon, consequent famine and migration to densely populated cities in search of work, creating ideal conditions for the spread of a respiratory infection. At least 12 million people died, about 5 per cent of the population, and there are vivid descriptions of rivers swollen with dead bodies because of the lack of firewood for cremation.

Mahatma Gandhi, then forty-nine years old, was infected. He recovered, but lost his daughter-in-law and grandchild to the disease. The healthcare system in the country was unable to meet the demands of the disease, and people continued to suffer. The misery, loss of life and economic impact led to an increase in anti-British sentiment.

The year 1918 did not mark the end of influenza pandemics; many influenza viruses have emerged and spread across the world since then, despite the availability of vaccines, but fortunately none have had as deadly an impact, including the latest H1N1 swine flu, which first appeared in Mexico in 2009.

Why Do New Infectious Agents Emerge and Spread?

New diseases seem to appear every few years among humans, and old diseases that were thought to have been controlled or gone reappear. There are many reasons why infectious diseases emerge, but recently the pace at which infectious diseases have affected humans around the world has accelerated, with about fifty new or re-emerging agents described since the 1970s. The reasons are manifold. People travel further and more often, there are several modes of transport, and it is possible for an infected person to carry her or his infecting bug to almost any major city in the world within twenty-four hours. Cities are growing and becoming more crowded, so contact between people is more frequent and lasts longer, which makes it easy for infections to spread. We are cutting down forests, so the contact between wild animals and humans is increasing, and viruses that may have been hidden away now have the chance to spread to a new host. The climate is changing with global warming, which means that the changes in temperature are allowing pathogens to survive for longer and spread to areas that were previously too cold for them. With battery farms and single-animal livestock operations, we are creating conditions conducive for the spread of infectious diseases in animals, birds and their handlers. The widespread use of antibiotics to prevent infections and as growth promoters can lead to the selection of drug-resistant superbugs, with potentially devastating consequences for humans.

Among new diseases that affect humans, a major contributor is the crossing of infectious agents from one species to another. These diseases, which come from non-human animals (or birds), are called zoonoses and they are quite common. Zoonoses made up about half of all new infectious agents in humans in the past half-century. Why does this happen? Much of the change in our encounters with animals of many kinds is driven by how we are changing and using ecosystems. As we encroach on forests and other animal habitats, settle in new areas, use new land for agriculture and animal husbandry, increase human population pressure, degrade land and travel more, we contribute to both enhancing the effects of climate change and increasing the burden of zoonotic infections. The greatest risk occurs where there is high growth of human populations and a significant overlap with wildlife populations. Hunting and mining activities are occupations at a higher risk of zoonotic infections. Deforestation is associated with increased chances of zoonotic infections, particularly in tropical areas, because both direct spread and spread through mosquitoes and other insects is possible. When land is cleared, we usually witness two phenomena—new human settlements emerge, which bring humans into contact with animals that lived there, and new habitats are created where insects breed and spread disease. Diseases spread by insects are called vector-borne, and many diseases such as dengue have increased greatly in the past few decades because of the degradation of the ecosystem and consequent increase in breeding habitats of mosquitoes.

There is an alphabet of zoonotic infections, and most of these diseases have become familiar to us in just the past few decades. A-AIDS, B-Bacillus anthracis, C-Chikungunya, D-Dengue, E-Enteroviruses, F-Filoviruses, G-German measles, H-Hantaan virus, I-Influenza, J-Japanese encephalitis virus, K-Kyasanur Forest disease virus, L-Lassa virus, M-MERS CoV, N-Nipah, O-Omsk haemorrhagic fever virus, P-Polio, Q-Q fever, R-Ross River virus, S-SARS-CoV, T-Tick-borne encephalitis virus, U-Usutu virus, V-Vibrio cholerae, W-West Nile virus, X-, Y-Yellow fever virus, Z-Zika virus.

In addition to infectious diseases that emerge and affect humans due to spread from animals, there is also the possibility of deliberate introduction of infectious agents into humans, animals or even plants. Examples of such diseases that could be used as biological weapons include anthrax, a bacterium usually found in sheep and cattle, or tularemia, which affects rabbits but can also affect many other species, including domestic animals and humans.

The inevitability of pandemics

A pandemic occurs when an infectious agent enters humans and is able to spread easily among them. In most cases, this happens when either the pathogen is a new—that humans have not encountered before—or one that has changed so much that the immune system is unable to recognize it and prevent the infection and disease.

Scientists have been warning the world for several years that our changing environment is increasing the likelihood of pandemics, and in 2009, the world had the last pandemic (before COVID-19) which was due to the H1N1 virus. The H1N1, while fulfilling the two criteria of being an infection with a modified virus and of being one that spreads easily, actually caused mainly asymptomatic or mild infections, although many people at a higher risk of severe disease due to age, illness or other conditions died. Influenza viruses are usually at the top of the lists of pandemic threats, followed by coronaviruses.

There are several reasons why influenza viruses are the prototype for pandemic agents. Influenza viruses have a genome that is made of ribonucleic acid or RNA. When this is copied to make new daughter viruses, mistakes can be made. This is not the case in other viruses where the genome is made of deoxyribonucleic acid or the DNA viruses, which have a proofreading mechanism. Further, unlike most other viruses, influenza viruses carry their genes on eight strands of RNA, instead of one. This makes the exchange of genes easier when there are two influenza viruses that infect a single host, resulting in the creation of a new virus with different genes. When humans live closely with domestic animals, such as ducks, chickens or pigs, which have many influenza viruses of their own, the viruses can mix together in these animals and then spread to humans. For example, the 2009 H1N1 virus, known as the swine flu virus, has genes that have come from pigs, humans and birds.

Therefore, influenza viruses have the first requirement for pandemics—that of being different enough for the human immune system to not recognize them and thus not being able to protect itself against them. The second requirement is the ability to spread among humans. Among the influenza viruses that have infected humans recently, we have a story of contrasts based on the ability to spread. The H5N1 virus or bird flu has been observed in humans since the early 2000s, and kills about half the people it infects. Fortunately for us, this virus so far does not spread very easily among humans, so most, though not all, infections have been because of the virus jumping from birds to humans. On the other hand, the 2009 H1N1 virus spread around the world in a few months, mainly because of humans travelling by air and carrying the virus. Again, fortunately for us, this virus was not as deadly as the H5N1 virus. But it is possible, even likely, that a virus as deadly as H5N1 and which spreads as easily as H1N1 will emerge—we just do not know when.

Making predictions requires not only communicating the likelihood of an event, but also its scale and its timing, and this is hard. There need to be a balance between unnecessary alarm and the danger of complacency and lack of preparedness. For infectious diseases, scientists have developed risk maps that show areas of the world that are likely to be sites where diseases could emerge and cause local or larger outbreaks.

With climate change, it seems inevitable that new infectious diseases will continue to be a significant risk to human health, and we need to think about how to deal better with them not only by reducing the chances of such emergence but also by building the ability to detect, track and manage potential threats.

2

COVID-19: A Pandemic, Not Just a Seasonal Flu

As cases of COVID-19 surged in India, a news reporter asked a woman in a remote village whether she had seen the coronavirus. The woman answered in the local dialect that the coronavirus is red and yellow in colour and about the size of a cricket ball. Images of SARS-CoV-2 have been flashing non-stop across every screen on every news channel for months, and have carried the coloured reconstruction of the virus to every corner of the country.

We know that viruses are smaller than bacteria and definitely cannot be seen without the help of a very powerful microscope, but the image and the name of the coronavirus are everywhere. We have auto-rickshaws remodelled as viruses, moving around towns and cities spreading the message of the need for caution. Television, radio and newspapers are paralleled by Kathakali performances and clever cartoons that are shared on WhatsApp, warning us all about the virus and what we should and should not do.

This advice is valuable, but understanding why we are given such advice is even more valuable. Coronaviruses, like other viruses and other micro-organisms, interact with their hosts in well-defined ways.

Humans and Microorganisms: Casual and causal relationships

Wherever in nature we find humans (for that matter, wherever we find animals or birds or insects), we find microorganisms. We have an intimate relationship with bacteria, viruses and fungi that have adapted to living with, in and on us. These microorganisms which we acquire at or shortly after birth very rarely cause any kind of harm, and in many ways are very beneficial to animals and human beings, breaking down cellulose in the gut and producing important vitamins. This kind of relationship between two living organisms is called symbiosis (meaning 'living together'), and symbiosis can benefit both or at least one partner, without any harm to the other. But once in a while we encounter a relationship with a microorganism, where one partner benefits and the other is harmed; here, the partner that benefits is the pathogen ('causing disease'), while the one that is harmed is the host.

All viruses require a host cell to replicate, because they cannot reproduce without using the machinery of the host. But even with this requirement, many viruses reproduce at such a low rate that host cells are not damaged a lot, and we do not even notice the viral infection. These are called inapparent infections. However, the entry of some viruses and their replication in the host can result in disease in a number of ways. A viral infection can result in illness because that particular virus may be recognized by the immune system which tries to get rid of it. Illness could also be caused if host cells are killed by a virus that enters the body and multiplies or if the virus produces substances that can damage cells or if the host immune system tries to kill the virus-infected cells, but in the process also causes damage to the host cells.

Viral Structure, Entry and Reproduction

Peter Medawar in 1977 called viruses 'a piece of bad news wrapped up in protein'. While that is true of the structure of viruses, not all viruses result in illness. Many factors influence whether a viral infection results in illness or not. Viruses infect the host through multiple routes. Viruses that infect the gut and cause diseases are usually brought in by food and water, or sometimes by close contact. Respiratory viruses come in through the nose and mouth or through contact (i.e., a person touches a surface and then his/her face). Some viruses enter through the parenteral ('outside the intestine') route, which could be via sexually transmitted infections or those acquired through injections or blood transfusions, for instance, HIV or hepatitis B.

Once a virus enters the human body, it infects the cells of its target organ, the gut, lungs, liver, brain, immune cells or other cells. To infect the host cell, the virus has to find a way to stick to it and then finally find its way inside. Usually the virus does this by having a protein on its surface which recognizes a corresponding protein (termed receptors) on the surface of the host cell. The viral protein and host cell protein then adhere to each other and that process of sticking together sparks a series of reactions in the host which permit the virus to get itself fully or partially inside the host cell. Many viruses have an envelope or outer coating which is usually discarded outside the host as it enters the cell, while there are others, like bacteriophages, which only send the genetic material into the host cell.

Viral genetic material may consist of RNA or DNA, which stores the genetic information that underpins all life. The viral genome may be one strand which carries information for many proteins as in SARS-CoV-2, or may be many strands as in the influenza virus. The viral genome is wrapped in one or more layers of proteins, and for some viruses, there is also an outer envelope which can contain lipid and proteins. Viruses can be of many shapes and sizes, from the 20-nanometre adeno-associated viruses to the 500-plus-nanometre megavirus, from the bullet-shaped rabies virus, or the distinctive adenovirus which looks like a satellite, complete with fibres extending from the penton corners, to the sun-shaped coronaviruses.

No matter what the shape, size or nuclear material of the virus, all viruses need to eventually get the host cell to copy their genetic information to make new DNA or RNA and also make the proteins that constitute its protein shell or capsid. Once the copies of the genome and the proteins are made, they can either be assembled inside the host cell, or be budded off from the host with the final assembly happening at the point of exit. Frequently, but not always, there are so many copies of the virus made in the host cell that the cell bursts to release the new viruses, which can then go on to infect other host cells, or be let out of the body, as in the case of respiratory or gut viruses, through sneezing or diarrhoea, to infect other hosts.

The Coronaviruses

Coronaviruses are a large group of RNA viruses that cause illness in humans, animals and birds. In cattle, they cause diarrhoea and in mice they infect the liver and the brain. In humans and birds, coronaviruses cause respiratory infections, which can range from mild to fatal. Coronaviruses have 26,000 to 32,000 bases of RNA which carry the sequence for about thirty proteins, making these viruses large and complex. The genome is surrounded by a protein shell, the nucleocapsid, and then by an envelope. All coronaviruses have spikes which project outwards from the surface and give the viruses an image that looks like the points of a crown under the electron microscope, hence the name 'corona'.

Coronaviruses were first discovered in birds in the 1920s, causing acute infections resulting in gasping in chickens. It was almost forty years later that the first coronavirus in humans as found in people with colds in the UK and the US. Their characteristic structure was first seen under the electron microscope in 1967 by June Almeida at the St Thomas' Hospital in London. There are four coronaviruses known to cause common cold in humans, with the last of these four viruses being identified in Hong Kong in 2004.

In 2003, for the first time, a coronavirus was found to cause severe respiratory disease. The disease caused by this virus was known as Severe Acute Respiratory Syndrome or SARS. Now known as SARS-CoV, the virus was first noticed when there was an increase in the number of cases in Hong Kong. It then spread to many other parts of the world. Despite the infectiousness and severity of the disease, it was soon recognized that the disease spread could be controlled by isolating patients and making sure that the hospital staff looking after patients did not get infected. Work on developing a vaccine started at the time. However, by testing people with respiratory symptoms, quickly isolating them and taking precautions to prevent infection, the number of infected people quickly declined and the disease finally disappeared. By 2004, almost 8000 people had been infected and about 9 per cent of them had died.

There was a lot of speculation about where the virus had come from, and investigations of wet markets where animals and birds were sold were conducted. The SARS-CoV was found in palm civets in Guangdong, China. Further surveys showed that the virus could be present in raccoons, ferrets and bats. It is now believed that the virus may have originated in bats, spread to civets and then to humans.

In September 2012, a new coronavirus causing severe respiratory disease was identified in a patient in Saudi Arabia. Over the next few months, occasional cases continued to be reported. While the source was unknown, it was thought that the virus did not spread from person to person. This was proved to be wrong when healthcare workers contracted the infection from patients in France and South Korea. Further research showed that the virus, now called Middle

East Respiratory Syndrome-Coronavirus (MERS-CoV), was found in camels and bats. It is now believed that the MERS-CoV spreads from bats to camels, and camels pass it on to humans. These introductions from camels to humans are not rare, but fortunately, the spread between humans does not often happen with good care and nursing. So far, about 2400 people have been infected and more than one-third of them have died.

SARS-CoV-2

At the end of December 2019, health authorities in Wuhan reported a cluster of respiratory infections. This was picked up and reported in the Chinese media and then by ProMED, the Program for Monitoring Emerging Diseases, run by the International Society for Infectious Diseases, which reported that an 'urgent notice on the treatment of pneumonia of unknown cause' had been issued by the medical administration of the Wuhan Municipal Health Commission. As the news spread around the world, the WHO followed up with China, and new information began to emerge every day. First, the cases appeared to be linked to the Huanan seafood wholesale market, which was shut down. The virus was rapidly identified as a coronavirus and by 11 January 2020, Chinese scientists and their Australian collaborators had released the first complete genomic sequence of the virus, showing that it was related to SARS-CoV.

The virus was initially called the 2019 novel Coronavirus or 2019-nCoV. On 11 February 2020, it was officially named the Severe Acute Respiratory Syndrome Coronavirus-2

(SARS-CoV-2). Viruses are named by the virus study groups of the International Committee on Taxonomy of Viruses (ICTV), while diseases are officially named by the WHO in the International Classification of Diseases (ICD). The WHO announced 'COVID-19' as the name of this new disease, where 'CO' stands for corona, 'VI' for virus and 'D' for disease. The numerical 19 indicated the year 2019, in which the disease was first reported. This is not the first time that the disease and the virus have had different names. HIV is the virus that causes Acquired Immunodeficiency Sydrome or AIDS. People often know the name of a disease, but not the name of the virus that causes it.

After the virus emerged in Wuhan, the number of infections started climbing rapidly. At first, it was not clear whether all the cases were originating in animals, but soon it was shown that human-to-human spread was taking place, and by the third week of January 2020, it was clear that the disease was spreading well beyond Wuhan and China. The WHO declared the outbreak as a 'public health emergency of international concern' (PHEIC) on 30 January 2020. It was the sixth time that a disease was declared a PHEIC by the WHO in the last thirteen years. COVID-19 was declared a pandemic on 11 March 2020.

How is SARS-CoV-2 different from the other coronaviruses?

All coronaviruses cause respiratory infections in humans. In the case of humans, four coronaviruses cause symptoms of common cold, and the infections are mild, but from what is known so far, the protection after infection does not last very long, so re-infection with the same coronavirus is a possibility. With SARS and MERS, the respiratory infection is severe: one in every eleven people with confirmed infection with SARS died (the disease has not been reported after 2004), and one in three people infected with MERS die. But with SARS and MERS, the spread to other humans, while it happens, is not like the infection and spread that we see with SARS-CoV-2.

SARS caused lower respiratory tract infection with pneumonia, but it was not able to infect the upper airway so human-to-human spread was less. Further, the SARS virus was released by the infected person only after they were sick, unlike what we are seeing with SARS-CoV-2. SARS-CoV-2 infects the nose and the upper respiratory tract, so coughing and sneezing easily spreads the infection. Also, with SARS-CoV-2, an infected person can be infectious for two to three days before they become sick. Since the infected people do not know that they are infected, they go around with their usual business and can easily infect others. It is also possible for people to be infected without ever knowing it, if they remain asymptomatic throughout. Infection with SARS-CoV-2 seems to have a very wide range and an entire spectrum, from people who never know that they were infected to those who become very sick and die. Even today, it is still not clear how many people are infected and have no illness, but it is estimated to be between 25 to 40 per cent of the total infections in any setting.

SARS-CoV-2 also differs from SARS and MERS in the way it infects not just the respiratory system and the gut, but also affects the heart, brain, and other organs. It was initially found that, like SARS, SARS-CoV-2 used the spike protein on its surface to bind to a protein on the surface of the host cell, called the angiotensin-converting enzyme 2 (ACE2), in order to enter the host cell. This receptor is found on many kinds of cell, and the SARS-CoV-2 binds well to it, much better than SARS does, which also happens to use the same protein. The spike protein is then primed by another protein called TMPRSS-2, which finally allows the virus to enter the cell.

Recent data has shown that SARS-CoV-2 uses another protein called neuropilin-1 as well. This protein has the ability to bind to more than one receptor on host cells which gives SARS-CoV-2 an advantage in rapid spread since it can infect more cells and easily. As new data emerges about the ways in which the virus gets into cells, we also have more options to find drugs that can help stop the infection by blocking the entry of the virus.

How does SARS CoV2 spread?

The virus spreads in many ways—through direct person-to-person contact, indirect contact, large droplet sprays, aerosols or a combination of these. Although the virus is also excreted in the feces, the feco-oral transmission of the disease is not considered to be significant. The main route is through respiratory droplets or aerosols, released when an infected person coughs, sneezes or talks. Moreover, droplets generated in such a way also land on surfaces, where the virus can survive. Infection can happen if a person touches an infected surface and then touches his or her eyes, nose or mouth.

There has been a lot of discussion about the size of the droplets or particles, which helps in deciding the distance that we should maintain between people, what the ventilation should be like and how long to spend with people if we want to limit the spread of infection. Much of the early discussion was based on studies of other viruses, particularly what was known about influenza, but over the past few months, many researchers who specialize in the physics of particles and liquids have provided new and useful data to help public health experts to come up with preventive measures.

In describing the spread of the virus, epidemiologists who study diseases in populations often use the basic reproduction number, R naught or R_0, which is the number of people to whom one infected person can spread the disease, assuming that no one has any protection from being infected. While this is a useful concept to understand how infectious a pathogen is (for instance, the measles virus is five times more infectious than SARS-CoV-2), the spread of disease can be influenced by many other factors. In addition, there are 'superspreading' events which we will describe later.

Respiratory droplets come from the nose or mouth when a person talks (more when one is loud and less when whispering), coughs or sneezes. The droplets can be of a range of sizes. The smaller particles remain suspended in air for a long time and accumulate in a room if there is no ventilation, while the large ones fall quickly to the ground or any lower surface. There are studies which show that a single cough can produce up to 100,000 droplets and could put 200,000,000 (two hundred million) virus particles into the air. Since experiments on animals indicate that we need less than 1000 particles for an infection with SARS-CoV-2, it is clear why this infection can be easily passed on from person to person.

Incubation Period

The time between getting infected and the first appearance of symptoms of the disease is called the incubation period. The incubation period for COVID-19 ranges from one to fourteen days. The most common or the median incubation period is about five days. For SARS-CoV-2, unlike many other viruses, the time when an infected person becomes infectious (because the virus has to multiply enough to be able to spread easily), is two or three days before they become symptomatic. In people who never develop symptoms, we know that they can spread disease because they have a lot of virus when they are tested, but we do not know for how long. For people who have symptoms, they are usually infectious for about one week after their symptoms start.

High-risk Groups

People of all ages can be infected, but those who are over the age of sixty are at higher risk of moderate to severe disease. People with underlying pre-existing medical conditions such as obesity, diabetes, hypertension, cardiac disease, chronic lung disease, cerebrovascular disease, chronic kidney disease, immune suppression and cancer are likely to have more severe disease and can die. Other conditions that increase the risk of serious illness include smoking, asthma, liver disease and being overweight.

Men are at a higher risk than women of suffering from severe disease. Pregnant women with COVID-19 have been shown to have a slightly higher chance of pre-term birth, but it is not clear whether this is because the women were very sick and therefore had their babies born too soon or whether the infection leads to pre-term labour. Most children have asymptomatic or mild infections, but occasional severe disease among children has been reported. A few children have been reported with an inflammatory illness that affects multiple organs resulting in fever, abdominal pain and other symptoms. This syndrome, regarded as unique for COVID-19, is known as multi-system inflammatory syndrome in children and is being better understood know. It can happen even after the child has recovered from the infection. It is not common, but has been reported from many countries.

Clinical symptoms in COVID-19

People with COVID-19 may have no symptoms or be critically ill. Generally, they can be grouped into well-defined categories, but it is important to remember that this may change with time. Infections can be of the following types:

- *Asymptomatic or Presymptomatic*: The infected in this category have tested positive for SARS-CoV-2 (that is, a nucleic acid amplification test or an antigen test), but they have no symptoms that are suggestive of infection with COVID-19. People who do not ever develop illness are asymptomatic, while those who developed illness later were presymptomatic at the time they were tested.

- *Mild*: People grouped under the mild illness category have fever, cough, sore throat, tiredness, headache, muscle pain, nausea, vomiting, diarrhoea, loss of taste and smell, but do not have shortness of breath, and their oxygen saturation is normal. Other viral infections also result in similar symptoms, but the loss of taste and smell seems to be greater in SARS-CoV-2 infections.

- *Moderate*: These are cases with difficulty in breathing or abnormal X-rays or CT scans and a fall in oxygen level (less than 94 per cent). They may require supplemental oxygen. In these patients, the oxygen levels in the blood are measured using a pulse oximeter. It is a small device that shows the oxygen level when it is clipped on a finger. This device is now routinely used to assess oxygen saturation at the facility level as well as for most other patients including those in home isolation (for early identification of illness becoming worse).

- *Severe*: Individuals who have low oxygen levels, rapid breathing and significant lung damage. They need high-flow oxygen, non-invasive ventilation and other medical interventions such as proning.

- *Critical*: Individuals who have respiratory failure, septic shock and/or multiple organ dysfunction. Patients in this category need devices to assist them in breathing and oxygenation. This group of patients will need ICU care, and possibly ventilators.

The COVID-19 management guidelines in India have combined the severe and critical types into one category (severe) to simplify the management protocol.

There are other non-specific symptoms. Older people and immune-suppressed patients may not have fever, but they may show symptoms like reduced alertness, reduced mobility, diarrhoea, loss of appetite or delirium. These symptoms may also be present in healthy persons without fever. Children may not report fever or cough as frequently as adults.

Studies across the world suggest[1] that of all the symptomatic cases, about 80 to 85 per cent of patients will be in the mild and moderate categories, while 10 to 18 per cent will be in the severe category, and 2 to 5 per cent may be critical.

In addition to respiratory symptoms and the subsequent scarring of the lungs, it is now recognized that this disease can cause sepsis and septic shock, multi-organ failure, including acute kidney injury and cardiac injury. This virus can directly attack other organs, it can cause inflammation of blood vessels, promote clotting in the blood, alter our immune mechanism and promote an enhanced inflammatory response in our body which is called a 'cytokine storm', or cytokine release syndrome, and this may damage many organs. This does not happen in all infected people, but in some it can have serious consequences, and thus COVID-19 is now considered a 'systemic disease' that can affect not just the lungs, but the brain, kidneys,

---

[1] Available at https://www.who.int/docs/default-source/coronaviruse/risk-comms-updates/update-36-long-term-symptoms.pdf?sfvrsn=5d3789a6_2.

intestines, skin, liver as well as many other organs, particularly the circulatory system.

At times, in some people, the clotting of blood can affect the blood vessels in the brain, leading to stroke and seizures. In most, the lung is the primary organ involved. Due to multiple factors, such as viral pneumonia and the clotting of vessels in the lungs, the oxygen level in the body falls as the affected lung is not able to extract oxygen from the air and deliver it to the blood. Often the patient does not realize that his or her oxygen level is low, and they don't complain of any breathing difficulty. This odd phenomenon has been termed 'happy hypoxia' (hypoxia meaning low oxygen). Many severely ill patients need high-flow oxygen or ventilator support to maintain an optimum oxygen level or just to be able to breathe. These patients need ICU care and may develop further complications related to being on a ventilator such as secondary bacterial pneumonia and septic shock. This can increase mortality. Besides lung or heart failure, acute kidney injury and liver dysfunction can occur in those who have serious illness. Therefore, what really helps to save lives in the absence of definitive treatment is good supportive care. Treatment directed at preventing not just complications related to the viral infection but also other complications that can occur while the body recovers and fights the virus has helped save lives in the ICU.

In addition to the initial SARS-CoV2 infection which can be mild to moderate or severe, we are also finding that patients who have recovered can continue to have lingering symptoms. This has been termed long-Covid or post-Covid syndrome. Lingering symptoms are more common in those patients who required hospitalization, but are also reported by those who managed their infection at home. In most individuals the symptoms are usually mild and range from fatigue, joint pain, body ache and anxiety to chest pain, breathlessness, and headache. These usually go away within six to eight weeks.

Some COVID-19 patients, the unfortunate few, may have significant organ damage and this may affect their quality of life for a long time. Patients with lung involvement may develop permanent damage to the lung tissues, leading to scarring in the lung. However, scarring in the lung does not cause too much of a breathing problem because lungs have significant reserve, but in some cases the damage is greater and home oxygen support is needed. The heart muscles of some patients have also shown damage when imaging was done months after infection. This has happened even in young and healthy people who suffered from a mild form of the disease. What this means is that the long-term damage that COVID-19 can cause is hard to predict at this time. COVID-19 makes blood cells more likely to clump up together and form clots. Large clots or thrombi can cause heart attacks and strokes, but this is less common than small clots that block small blood vessels (capillaries) in the heart causing heart muscle damage. Blood clots also affect other organs such as the lungs, legs, liver and kidneys. COVID-19 can also weaken blood vessels, which contributes to potentially long-lasting problems with the liver and kidneys.

Apart from the acute effect that COVID-19 can cause in the brain in the form of stroke, seizures or encephalitis, it can also cause long-term effects. Many people report a 'brain fog', a condition where they are forgetful and are not able to comprehend what is happening. Many patients suffer from chronic fatigue syndrome, insomnia and exhaustion for months after recovering. They would need regular physiotherapy and caregiver support.

How Is Infection Diagnosed?

Everyone is now familiar with pictures of a person wearing a full body cover, mask, goggles and gloves, collecting specimens from the nose of a patient. However, in reality, many kinds of specimens can be used with varying levels of preference. The virus infects and multiplies in the upper and lower part of the respiratory tract. The best specimen for patients with severe illness is actually a washing of the lung through a bronchoscope, called bronchoalveolar lavage. For people with no or mild illness, the tests can be done on deep nasal or oral swabs, or even on saliva. Usually, specimens are collected by using special swabs, which can be tested directly by the rapid antigen test kits or sent to a laboratory for testing by RT-PCR. If the specimens are to be transported, then the swabs are put in a tube that contains a fluid called viral transport medium (VTM), which prevents the breakdown of the virus. The transport is usually done in iceboxes to preserve the virus.

To diagnose present infection, we have to show that the virus is there. This is done by looking for either the protein shell by tests that bind to the protein and then are seen as a colour signal (this can be seen in the widely used rapid antigen tests which look for the appearance of coloured lines on a membrane strip, or other tests that are done in a laboratory), or by looking for the RNA of the virus. To do the latter, the protein shell is broken apart, and the virus RNA is converted to DNA and copied millions of times using special enzymes. This copying, which is part of the polymerase chain reaction (PCR), makes it easy to detect whether the viral genes are present or not.

To diagnose past infection, we look for antibodies of different kinds, either to the spike or to the proteins in the shell. There are different kinds of antibodies, and most available tests are for IgG, with a few for IgA and IgM antibodies. The presence of antibodies shows that viral infection has happened, but in 10 to 20 per cent of the people antibodies may not be found even after confirmed infection. Usually, the more severe the disease, the greater the percentage of people who have antibodies, but the tests must be done about four weeks after the RT-PCR, as antibodies may decrease after a few months.

What Is the Treatment?

There is currently no proven treatment; however, a few experimental therapies are approved (more details in chapter 7).

Conclusion

SARS-CoV-2 is part of a large family of viruses that infect many species around the world. In less than a year, SARS-CoV-2 made the jump from an unknown animal species to humans in China and then spread around the world. This virus is very infectious because it has the unique ability to bind easily and strongly to human lung cells and the cells in other organs of the body. Infection with the virus results in a range of symptoms from no disease to mild disease to a severe and fatal disease. The latter is experienced particularly by people who have pre-existing health conditions. Initially, opinions varied between this being a killer virus to being no worse than a bad flu. We know now that most infections resolve, but a small proportion of people continue to have serious issues after the acute infection is over. This is not the flu!

Section II

Mounting a Response

3

Preparedness: Barely a Choice

The flying time from Wuhan, China, to Kochi, India, is 8 hours and 45 minutes. However, it took a twenty-three-year-old medical student from Kerala—studying in Wuhan University—five days and a few hours to reach his home in Kasaragod district (approximately 350 kilometres from Kochi).

On 22 January 2020, he took a taxi from Wuhan University to the city railway station, where he boarded a train and reached Guangzhou on 23 January. In Guangzhou, he stayed with sixteen other students from India till 25 January. He took a flight from Guangzhou to Kolkata on 25 January. On the same day, he took another flight from Kolkata to Bengaluru, then a taxi to his hotel room in Bengaluru, where he stayed overnight. On 26 January, he boarded a flight from Bengaluru to arrive in Kochi. Then, he travelled by a taxi from Kochi airport to Aluva railway station and boarded a train to Kasaragod. He deboarded at the very next station, Angamaly, due to non-availability of a sleeper berth. From

Angamaly station, he took an autorickshaw to a hotel where he stayed overnight. On 27 January, he took a public bus from the hotel back to Aluva railway station and boarded a train for Kanhangad. He travelled in a private vehicle along with two other people and reached home in Kasaragod, on the night of 27 January. He wore a mask from Wuhan till Kolkata but not thereafter. He had no symptoms of the disease when he reached home.

On the third day of his arrival, he developed symptoms of upper respiratory tract infection. He was admitted to the isolation ward of the district hospital. He tested positive as one of the first three COVID-19 cases reported from India. District officials estimated that during his journey, he was exposed to 189 primary or direct contacts and 305 secondary contacts. All of them were at potential risk. This single event could have been enough for the outbreak of 2019-nCoV (as it was named then) in India.

Cautious Start and Concerned People

Three weeks before this student left Wuhan, health authorities in China had alerted the WHO about a new type of respiratory illness, caused by the virus, which was not reported earlier. Thereafter, cases had been reported from Thailand, South Korea and Japan. There were reports of many cases emerging from different parts of Wuhan and other provinces in China.

India was closely monitoring these developments. The ministry of health and family welfare (MoHFW), Government of India, issued an advisory on 17 January 2020. People returning from China and a few other countries began to be screened at select airports from 18 January 2020. The Joint Monitoring Group (JMG) in the MoHFW was activated and experts began keeping track of the situation and working on developing protocols to strengthen infrastructure for health staff to respond to the emerging scenario.

Testing for 2019-nCoV was initiated on 22 January 2020 at the National Institute of Virology (NIV) in Pune. Around 24 January 2020, when news of the lockdown in Wuhan emerged, the need for more preventive interventions and COVID-19 testing in India was perceived. To respond to public queries and track the situation, a 24x7 call centre was set up at the National Centre for Disease Control (NCDC) in New Delhi.

While everyone was receiving sporadic news of the outbreak in China, the Government of India formed a few teams comprising public health experts, clinicians and microbiologists to visit and assess the levels of preparedness of seven airports which had begun screening people returning to India.

On 30 January 2020, the WHO designated the outbreak as public health emergency of international concern (PHEIC). On the same day, news came that Russia and China had already started working on a vaccine. In the afternoon of the same day, India's first case of COVID-19—a student, who had returned from Wuhan—was reported from Thrissur, Kerala.

The Real Airlift

Wuhan in China was in lockdown. Indian students residing there wanted to come back. Foreign ministry officials in India and China started discussions on airlifting them. The first Air India flight landed in Wuhan on 31 January 2020. A team of doctors and nurses from leading government institutes were accompanying the aircraft crew. They had limited information about the various medical aspects. They knew that the disease was highly contagious. However, they had little or no experience of dealing with the disease and most of them had never donned PPE.

On the way to Wuhan, the crew and medical team on-board brainstormed for situations which could arise and how to respond to them in real time. What if someone had crossed the first checkpoint and was found symptomatic during the second screening by the Indian crew? How was the biomedical waste to be disposed? Finally, over 600 students landed in Delhi in two days and the next task was to put them in quarantine.

New Addition to the Public Vocabulary: 'Quarantine'

With the evacuation from Wuhan, the word 'quarantine' came into vogue. In fact, it was just the beginning of the entry of many new public health and medicine terms into daily life. The word dates back to the fourteenth century with the outbreak of the Black Death in Europe. 'Quarantine' literally means 'space of forty days' and originated from the city of Venice which had enforced the policy of holding ships coming from plague-stricken countries at the port for forty days. This was enforced even when people on the ship had no symptoms. The city authorities had realized that people might initially be healthy (the incubation period which refers to the time lag, usually in days, from the person getting the infection to the appearance of the initial clinical symptoms) and there was no way to be sure whether someone was infected or not. The best way to stop the spread of disease was to quarantine people, even if healthy, for forty days.

The purpose of quarantine is to prevent the transmission of an infectious or contagious disease from potentially infected persons to healthy persons, especially during the incubation period. It differs from isolation in that the latter refers to segregation of people with clinical symptoms. Thus, quarantine is meant for healthy people who may or may not be infected, while isolation addresses those who have developed symptoms and are either suspected or confirmed to be infected.

The evacuees from Wuhan had to be either quarantined or isolated. They were to be screened again on arrival and two quarantine facilities were set up to house them. Those with symptoms were to be sent to the identified isolation facilities established at designated hospitals.

The Indian Army was entrusted with the responsibility of setting up a quarantine facility in Manesar (Haryana) to house students and other people who were brought back to India. An existing structure was converted into the facility for the purpose. It had administrative areas, arrangement for accommodation as well as medical facilities. Barracks and sectors were created in the accommodation area. Each sector could accommodate approximately fifty people. Furthermore, there were barracks for smaller groups. People were allowed to interact only with people in their own barracks and that too from a safe distance.

The evacuees were screened by a joint medical team comprising the Armed Forces Medical Services (AFMS) and the Airport Health Organization (APHO) under Directorate General of Health Services (DGHS). They were arranged into three groups. The first group had suspected cases (those who had fever, cough or respiratory distress). The second group comprised people who had no symptoms but had come into contact with a person with symptoms or visited an animal or seafood market or even a health facility in China in the two weeks preceding their return to India. The third group included 'non-contact individuals'.

All 'suspect' cases were sent to the isolation ward at the Army Research and Referral Hospital in Delhi. The others were sent to quarantine centres either in Manesar or at the facility run by the Indo-Tibetan Border Police in Chhawla in Najafgarh, Delhi. The quarantine centre in Manesar was run by a medical officer in-charge along with experts on medicine, nursing officers, at least one female woman medical officer and a nursing assistant. For the first time, the entire staff posted at these two facilities wore PPE, including masks, eye shields, shoe covers, gowns and gloves. People in quarantine were mandatorily required to wear a 'three-layered surgical mask' throughout the stay. No one housed in the facility, whether resident or staff, was allowed to leave unless they had a medical emergency.

At the end of the fourteen-day quarantine period, people were tested for COVID-19 and discharged only when they tested negative. None of the evacuees was found positive. On discharge, each was given a health certificate and detailed documentation was sent to state and district surveillance officers.

Being Prepared: The Kerala Experience

The state of Kerala addressed the virus with foresight. It had identified and efficiently handled the Nipah virus outbreak in 2018 and 2019. During that period, the state government had created isolation wards, trained health staff, activated a surveillance system and strengthened the public health network in every district. The state understood the concepts of isolation and quarantine well.

Being adequately prepared is half the battle won in pandemics. The experience gave Kerala a distinct advantage. The first case was confirmed from Thrissur district. The female student was isolated and her contacts quarantined. Two other cases were reported from Alappuzha and Kasaragod districts. Field staff was put on alert and the state health machinery went into overdrive. The cases were moved to isolation wards in district hospitals and their contacts—nearly 1000 people—were traced and asked to self-quarantine.

The Rapid Response Centre (RRC) in the state capital was activated and thereafter it met twice a day, with the state's health minister too participating in the meetings. The state government had formed eighteen expert groups on various thematic areas such as home quarantine, contact tracing, isolation, logistics and training. The availability of isolation beds, hospital beds and facilities in private sector was tracked on a regular basis. Public health officials and medical officers from the primary health centres (PHCs) were coordinating every development with the district administration. A panchayat secretary was assigned to every village to coordinate and monitor the outbreak at the grassroots.

Watchful and Alert

After the third case in Kerala, public health efforts were stepped up all across the country. Expert committees were set up in a number of states, with the MoHFW's Joint Monitoring Group (JMG) keeping a close eye on the evolving situation. Standard protocols were being developed, airport screening was enhanced, samples from suspected cases were being sent for laboratory testing and the numbers of testing laboratories were also being increased. By mid-February, the number of COVID-19 testing laboratories was increased to fifteen and one of the government laboratories was designated a global reference lab. The situation in India seemed to ease after 3 February and things seemed to be returning to normal. There were elections in some states. High-profile visits of heads of states followed. Conferences, meetings, offices and schools went on as usual.

Just when people were beginning to hope that India had been spared the brunt of the virus, things took a turn for the worse by the end of February, with a spike in cases almost all over the world. The WHO raised the level of global risk to 'very high'. By the first week of March 2020, Delhi, Telangana and Rajasthan were beginning to report their first cases in quick succession.

On 2 March 2020, two cases were reported from Delhi and Hyderabad. The patients had travelled from Italy and Dubai, respectively. On that day, across the country, around thirty-seven people were put under isolation and 26,000 under home surveillance. At twenty-one airports, nearly 557,000 people had been screened. Nearly 3250 samples had tested positive. Globally, around 89,000 COVID-19 cases were reported with close to 3000 deaths. Most of these cases were in China, South Korea, Italy, Iran and Japan.

The staff on duty at the thirty-two-bed isolation facility at a leading hospital in Delhi, where the first Delhi case had been admitted, were advised to go for a fourteen-day home quarantine. People who came in contact with the patients from Delhi and Hyderabad were identified and traced. After returning from Italy, the patient from Delhi had reportedly organized a birthday party for his child in a leading hotel in Delhi. Children who came to the party later attended school in Noida. Some of the contacts of the first case were isolated while a few were quarantined, based on risk assessed. The school was shut for a week as a preventive measure. The story of the patient from Hyderabad was similar to that of Delhi. On arriving at Bengaluru from Dubai, he took a private bus to Hyderabad, where he was hospitalized, tested and found positive. In the end, nearly eighty-eight contacts, including twenty-seven people from the bus, his flatmate and twenty-five colleagues were screened.

In the days to follow, cases began to be reported in large numbers. State governments started to form task forces to deal with the situation. New isolation wards were created and existing ones revamped. Plans were put in place on a war footing to increase the number of testing facilities, isolation beds and additional facilities as well as to procure N95 masks.

Simple Public Health Tools to Fight the Big Challenge

Tools and approaches deployed to prevent the spread of the disease included contact tracing, testing and isolation (or quarantine). Though testing and quarantine were concepts people were aware of, albeit in the context of other diseases, contact tracing was something very few had heard of before the pandemic. It has proved to be among the most powerful tools to fight the virus (see Box 3.1).

Box 3.1 Steps Involved in Contact Tracing

- **Contact identification:** This involves the identification of every person who may have come in contact with a confirmed infected case before the latter tested positive for COVID-19.
- **Contact listing:** Once these contacts are identified, a list is prepared with addresses and contact details. Health workers start calling them or visiting them in person to check their health status. The level of risk is assessed and some are advised for testing. Those at relatively low exposure and risk are advised to undertake a fourteen-day home quarantine.
- **Contact follow-ups:** Regular follow-ups are made regarding their health conditions.

Contact tracing was very intensive in the initial stages of the outbreak. On an average, for every case detected, around 50 to 150 contacts were identified and traced. In a few states the services of call centres were utilized to follow up with the contact twice a day. However, in many settings, frontline workers such as Accredited Social Health Activist (ASHA) and Anganwadi workers (AWW) visited households to trace contacts and then follow up regularly. They have been part of the government system for decades, but until the pandemic was declared, few people had heard of them.

It Is a Pandemic

On 11 March 2020, the WHO declared COVID-19 a pandemic. Soon after, the Indian government made a few decisions to halt the spread of the virus. International flights to and from India were stopped. State governments started to impose various types of curbs. On the same day, the Union government advised the state governments to invoke Section 2 of the Epidemic Diseases Act, 1897. Later, the Disaster Management Act, 2005, was also enforced.

Globally, countries started enforcing various versions of lockdowns. Norway enforced a lockdown on 12 March 2020. In the days to follow, many countries, including Denmark, Poland, Spain, France, Belgium and Germany, had imposed lockdowns. New Zealand closed its borders for all non-residents on 19 March and Australia on 20 March. The lockdown in the United Kingdom started on 23 March 2020. The situation in California and New York State of the USA was grave and they too ordered a form of lockdown, the 'stay at home' order.

In India, as a preventive measure, schools were already shut across a few states from the second and third week of March 2020. Many offices were shifting to a work-from-home mode. Policymakers and public health experts began deliberating on the next course of action. The stock market, in free fall over the previous weeks, had one of its biggest drops on 23 March 2020.

The prime minister of India convened a meeting of the leaders of South Asian Association for Regional Cooperation (SAARC) countries to collaborate about the pandemic. He made two addresses to the nation, including a voluntary call, the Janata Curfew, to stay at home on 22 March 2020. By 24 March 2020, the global numbers of COVID-19 cases had gone up to 407,000 cases and 18,250 deaths. India reported 536 cases and ten deaths. Nearly 2 billion people or one-fourth of the world's population was under lockdown, in nearly three dozen countries.

Time to Hit Back: The Hammer and Dance Theory

An article posted on the blogging site Medium by analyst Tomás Pueyo went viral. It argued for a 'hammer and dance' approach: a first, intense 'hammer' or heavy blow to stop the outbreak and then a sustained 'dance', multiple lighter measures, to contain the virus till there was a vaccine and/or other alternative solutions. The 'hammer' included strong measures such as lockdowns to cut the spread, recruitment of health personnel, building healthcare capacity, developing testing services and improving treatment services. This was proposed for three to seven weeks. Alongside, the 'dance' approach proposed 'testing, tracing, treating and isolating and quarantine', ban on large gatherings, public awareness on social distancing and hand hygiene. This analysis took into account several projections and infection trends on how an outbreak can be interrupted by containment efforts, such as compelling people to observe social distancing and shutting down schools, offices and public transport to ensure people are not physically close enough to infect each other.

Various 'disease modelling' tools were used to find the optimal way to respond to the pandemic. Model-based estimates started emanating from reputed institutes, which indicated that a 'do-nothing' approach could cost lives. Many in India, with its nearly 1.38 billion population, were unsure of what was going to happen next.

What Did Everyone Learn During This Period?

- **Outbreaks, epidemics, pandemics are a reality and being prepared is the best strategy.** Though pandemics are rare, outbreaks and epidemics keep happening in one or the other part of the world. Every country and health system needs to plan and prepare for such situations.

- **Preparedness, response and mitigation require multi-sectoral engagement and collaboration.** The level of preparedness and response to such settings is dependent upon multi-sectoral collaboration. High-level political leadership at both Union and state levels needs to be engaged in the process.

- **Health of the people across the world is interconnected.** The health situation in one country can affect all parts of the world and every citizen across the world. A coordinated and effective response by the world community and global leaders should be prioritized and implemented.

- **Health legislations are an integral part of an effective health system response.** The Epidemic Diseases Act, 1897, along with the Disaster Management Act, 2005, were used to mount the pandemic response. The context here was a pandemic, but even otherwise, effective health outcomes need coordinated legislative and regulatory interventions.

4

The Lockdown: Time to Respond

How much rush would one expect at a grocery store round the corner, late in the evening? A couple of customers maybe. In all likelihood, the shop owner would be busy counting the collection for the day. The support staff would be arranging the things lying outside back in their proper place on the racks. And then they will call it a day. However, on 24 March 2020, soon after 8.30 p.m., in many parts across urban India, there were long queues outside grocery stores. People were impatient to get inside the stores and those who did manage to find their way inside the shops, picked up whatever they could lay their hands on. That day, when the grocery stores finally closed, many of them looked like they had been plundered, albeit in a civilized manner. Empty shelves stared back at the owners. A short while ago, in an address to the nation, the prime minister had announced a countrywide lockdown for the next three weeks, which was going to be effective within a few hours.

A Virus That Paused the Olympics

By February and March 2020, the SARS-CoV-2 had already wreaked havoc in many countries including Spain and Italy. It was rapidly spreading in the USA. On 24 March 2020, a reputed international academic institute released model-based estimates, which projected 300 million COVID-19 cases and several thousand deaths in India, by the end of May 2020.[1]

On 25 March 2020, India had entered a nationwide lockdown. On the first day of the lockdown in India, far away in Tokyo, the International Olympic Committee (IOC) and the government of Japan were deliberating another major issue. Could the Olympics 2020 be held as per the schedule in July? Later that day, the IOC members agreed that it would not be possible to hold the Olympic Games this year. The countdown clock for the Tokyo 2020 Olympics was stopped. The summer Olympics had been cancelled thrice in the past: each time because of war. For the first time the Olympics had to be postponed because of a virus.

Lockdowns, Mass Self-Quarantine and 'Stay at Home' Orders

While no country or health system was ready for the challenges posed by the virus, a team at a reputed international academic

---

[1] Available at https://cddep.org/wp-content/uploads/2020/03/COVID19.indiasim.March23-2-eK.pdf.

institute had suggested lockdown as an immediate approach.[2] The proposed lockdown had a simple and twofold rationale: (a) slow the spread of virus and (b) accelerate the health system's readiness. Starting the second week of March 2020, a number of countries had adopted and implemented this approach as per their constitutional provisions. Most called it lockdown, a few called it 'voluntary mass quarantine' and a few others referred to it as 'stay at home' orders. Irrespective of what it was called, the objectives remained the same: to slow down the spread of the deadly virus and get health services ready.

Starting with the first lockdown from 25 March 2020, there were three more phases and the lockdown in India officially lasted for sixty-eight days. However, asking people to stay at home was not enough. The virus was already circulating and every now and then cases would emerge. More proactive responses were needed to control the spread. Initially, similar interventions were followed across the country and only essential services were allowed. In the subsequent phases, differential approaches were adopted to implement interventions and open up additional activities. The districts across India, based on number of cases and other parameters, were classified into red, yellow and green zones. Across the country, 'hotspots', that is, places where a majority of cases had emerged, were being identified. Similarly, in all districts, the approach of identifying containment zones was

---

[2] Available at https://www.imperial.ac.uk/media/imperial-college/medicine/sph/ide/gida-fellowships/Imperial-College-COVID19-NPI-modelling-16-03-2020.pdf.

being followed for more intensive interventions at the local level and strict lockdown measures were being adopted.

It was a period when a lot of data from within the country was analysed and reports from other countries studied to derive better epidemiological understanding[3] of the disease and its determinants.

Public Health Interventions for Pandemic Response

The epidemiologists (individuals, doctors, social scientists, disease modellers and many other graduates across streams, who are trained to understand the characteristics of disease-causing agents and their pattern of spread in the community) were busy determining the strategies to intervene to stop the spread. Two broad categories of interventions were proposed (see Box 4.1) that are detailed in the following sections.

Box 4.1 Public Health Interventions for COVID-19 Response

Public health interventions were needed for the entire population to fight the pandemic. These interventions were the following:

---

[3] The focus was on many aspects of epidemiology, with special attention on the descriptive epidemiology of those who were affected: what are the various time intervals such as from the time of getting infected to the development of symptoms and the places where the infections/cases were spreading.

(a) **Face masks, hand-washing and social/physical distancing:** Using face masks and covers, practising physical/social distancing and washing and sanitizing hands were identified as key interventions with the ability to reduce the spread of the virus. These are also referred to as non-pharmacological interventions. Though to be followed at individual and community levels, these required active interventions from the government, through Risk Communication and Community Engagement (RCCE). As part of the RCCE, the Union and state governments regularly communicated the risks and symptoms of the disease to the general public. Such communications were also essential to prevent misinformation and rumours.

(b) **Test, trace, treat, isolate:** COVID-19 testing, contact tracing, isolation of patients and ensuring the availability of quarantine facilities for those exposed to the infected people were the interventions to be implemented by the government. While use of face masks, hand-washing and social distancing were to be adopted by the people and supported by the government, this second set of interventions required to be implemented by the government, with active support from the people.

Handwashing: A Time-Tested Tool of Quarantine

Due to COVID-19, handwashing received attention once more after nearly 170 years. It may be unbelievable today, but nearly 200 years ago, doctors did not wear gloves for surgeries. Back then, nobody would doubt or question the cleanliness of the hands of doctors. Handwashing was not mandatory before surgical procedures, as it is today.

When a young Hungarian physician Ignaz Semmelweis joined the obstetrics department of Vienna Hospital in 1846, he found that the division where he was working had nearly sevenfold higher mortality than the other obstetrics division in the same hospital, which was staffed exclusively by midwives.[4] It was intriguing for him that doctors were less likely to save the lives of pregnant women than midwives. He investigated further and found that in the hospital, the physicians and medical students (who were part of the division where he worked) would start their day by conducting autopsies on women who had died the previous night or day. Once they were done with the autopsies, they would go into the labour rooms and conduct deliveries. While going from the autopsy room to the labour room, they would not clean their hands. Surgical gloves had not yet been invented, and all clinical procedures were done with bare hands.

In the other division, where nurses and midwives were in charge, the midwives did not do autopsies. They would start their day with deliveries. That was the key difference. It must be remembered that in those years the concept of germs was not known. The germ theory—that germs caused

---

[4] Available at https://theconversation.com/ignaz-semmelweis-the-doctor-who-discovered-the-disease-fighting-power-of-hand-washing-in-1847-135528.

diseases—emerged forty years later when Louis Pasteur proposed the concept in 1885.

Ignaz Semmelweis hypothesized that the physicians acquired something in their hands during the autopsy. He proposed and implemented a handwashing policy for all physicians and medical students before they entered the labour room. Within a year, the mortality was brought down to one-sixth of the former number and both units now had nearly similar mortality.

This was the first scientific proof that handwashing helped in preventing infection, though this did not immediately become popular among doctors. Once the concept of antisepsis by Joseph Lister and the germ theory proposed by Louis Pasteur were proven, the role of handwashing in infection prevention and control was recognized. Today, Ignaz Semmelweis is considered the father of hand hygiene and of infection control in hospitals. His work has saved millions of lives throughout the world.

Handwashing or 'washing' as it is commonly called by doctors and nurses across the world, has now become an essential procedure in modern health services. While handwashing became routine in healthcare, the role of handwashing and of hand hygiene in reducing disease spread has been slower in adoption.

Historically, the first use of handwashing for disease prevention was reported from the fourteenth century when some communities such as the Jews were found to have a lower death rate in the Black Death pandemic.[5] Many recognized

---

[5] Ibid.

that this was due to the custom and ritual of handwashing in these communities.

In public health, the role of soap and running water is widely recognized in preventing, controlling and reducing disease spread. There have been mass campaigns to adopt these habits, specially to prevent illnesses such as diarrhoea in children. Handwashing is considered a proven and among the most cost-effective public health interventions along with vaccination.

More recently, during SARS outbreak in 2002–04, the authorities in Hong Kong had advised the public to wash their hands to prevent the spread of the disease. During the COVID-19 pandemic, handwashing came to our rescue once again. Handwashing is one intervention that has the potential to reduce other infectious diseases not only in the days ahead but also in future, for instance, in the post-pandemic period.

Physical Distancing: Namaste the 'New Handshake'[6]

SARS-CoV-2 is known to spread through droplets generated from the mouth or nose of an infected person. The risk of transmission is directly proportionate to the number of droplets received, which also depends on the distance from the infected person. One metre is the minimum distance recommended between people; with any additional distance

---

[6] This was referred to as 'social distancing' in the early stages of the pandemic; however, the concept is more about maintaining physical distance.

maintained, the chances of infection go down. The Indian government has recommended a local adaptation of two *gaj* or six feet (1.8 metres) distancing.

The countrywide lockdown ensured that offices and schools remained closed as did the malls and restaurants. The suspension of sports events, the closure of public places and restrictions on the number of people who could attend public functions such as weddings and even funerals facilitated physical distancing. The lockdown included mass-scale operational approaches to ensure social distancing.

Masks and Face Covers: The Emblem of Pandemic Response

Masks were not mandatory for the entire public from the beginning of the pandemic. It emerged from the empirical understanding that the virus spread through droplets, and the use of face masks would reduce the transfer of droplets from one individual to another. Masks or face covers in public places soon became mandatory. From April 2020, many shops and places had strictly implemented a 'no mask, no entry' policy.

A few more weeks later, when it became clear that people could be infected yet show no symptoms themselves (the asymptomatic or presymptomatic ones), and that they could pass the infection to another without even realizing it, strict measures were implemented to enforce wearing of a mask at public places.

The masks served many purposes. One, masks reduced the chances of viruses on surfaces being carried by hands to one's eyes, nostrils or mouth by touching. Second, wearing a mask became a good reminder about the other preventive measures that one was supposed to follow. In the subsequent weeks, the role of masks changed from being primarily for self-protection to something that protects the wider community. Besides, people in many rural areas and slums do not have the luxury of having sufficient water and soap to wash hands. For them, masks and/or face cover were relatively low-cost and a measure that was easy to adhere to.

From Empirical to Evidence-Based Approach

The wearing of face masks, handwashing and physical distancing in the beginning were implemented based on empirical understanding. These had worked in the past in similar conditions and were likely to work here as well. Yet, soon more evidence emerged. A study published in *The Lancet* in June 2020, which had 172 studies from sixteen countries, found that all three interventions (face masks, physical distancing and handwashing) work.[7] A combination of the interventions works better than a single intervention. This study reported that the chances of infection were around 13 per cent when people maintained a distance of one metre. It got reduced to a fifth, that is

---

[7]   D. Chu, et al. 'Physical Distancing, Face Masks, and Eye Protection to Prevent Person-to-Person Transmission of SARS-CoV-2 and COVID-19: A Systematic Review and Meta-analysis'. *The Lancet*. 1 June 2020, https://doi.org/10.1016/S0140-6736(20)31142-9

2.6 per cent, when a distance of more than one metre was maintained. The study indicated that the risk halved with every extra metre of distance maintained, up to three metres.

Similarly, a number of studies and scientific evidence were published in the following months about the effectiveness of handwashing and of face masks in preventing the spread of the virus. Each one was partly effective and complementary together.

Breaking the Chain: Test, Trace and Isolate

In middle of April 2020, there was widespread panic when a food delivery person for a mobile-based application tested positive for COVID-19.[8] As per standard protocol, the delivery boy was admitted in an institutional isolation facility. A total of seventy-two families where he had delivered food before being tested positive were contacted and traced. They were advised to be in home quarantine for fourteen days. The local health staff regularly followed up with them. Seventeen other food delivery personnel who had come into contact with the COVID-19 positive patient were also tested and were admitted in institutional quarantine facilities, while their reports were awaited.[9] The restaurant where he worked

---

[8] Available at https://www.indiatoday.in/india/story/delhi-pizza-delivery-boy-tests-positive-for-coronavirus-1667501-2020-04-16.

[9] Isolation is for people who have tested positive. Quarantine is meant for healthy people who may have been exposed but their disease status is not yet known.

was temporarily closed. This is an example of how testing, tracing and quarantine/isolation worked. These were the public health interventions implemented by the government to break the chain of spread of SARS-CoV-2.

COVID-19 Testing

From the very beginning, COVID-19 testing was identified as one of the key approaches for pandemic response. The identification of suspected cases helped in early and immediate isolation of confirmed cases. Their contacts were traced for additional testing and quarantine. This was essential for preventing the spread of the virus. However, in the beginning, the number of laboratories with the capacity to conduct COVID-19 testing was limited. Moreover, the testing kits and reagents were not sufficiently available.

Recognizing the limited testing capacity and the other operational challenges, India adopted a calibrated strategy for COVID-19 testing. The approach has often been referred to as an approach of 'testing with purpose'. The COVID-19 testing strategy and protocols were developed and enforced as per the stage of the pandemic. Initially, only those with travel history to affected countries were being tested. Subsequently, the symptomatic contacts of confirmed cases were included. Gradually, testing was expanded to include symptomatic health workers, individuals in the hotspots who were symptomatic and the hospitalized severe acute respiratory illness (SARI) cases. Over a period of time, as the laboratory network expended, and more testing methods and approaches became available, the testing services were further expanded.[10]

Two broad categories of COVID-19 tests are currently being used: the antigen tests and antibody tests.

The antigen tests are conducted to detect the person with current COVID-19 infection. Initially, the only antigen test available was the RT-PCR test. This is a molecular test where part of the viral genome is identified and detected. The process makes it very sensitive and specific and is considered the gold standard in COVID-19 testing. However, RT-PCR requires laboratory set-up and the machines are expensive and not easily available in all cities. The process requires the samples to be collected, stored and transported to one of the designated laboratories for testing. In the early stage of the pandemic, these laboratories were not in the same district. Once the sample was collected, it would have to be sent to a different city and the entire process would take anywhere between five to seven days before the report became available. The other challenge with this strategy was that while waiting for the test report, if the concerned individual was not isolated, he or she could transmit the infection. Moreover, the need for isolating those undergoing testing was a deterrent as many people did not come forward for it. There was an urgent need for more laboratories and designated facilities to conduct tests and ensure the timely availability of reports. In June 2020,

---

[10] September 2020 onwards, a few states allowed walk-in testing or testing on request, where anyone could walk in and get the COVID-19 test done.

a rapid antigen test (RAT) was also approved in India. The benefit of RAT is that it can be done in a community setting, the results are available within fifteen to thirty minutes and the cost is relatively low. However, the limitation is that the sensitivity is relatively lower and it gives false negative reports (that is, a few individuals with infection may not be detected through RAT).

The second group is antibody tests. These tests are done to identify past infection. Most of these tests detect the IgG (immunoglobulin) type of antibody in a person. These antibodies are developed seven to fourteen days after the person is infected. These are used as a surveillance tool to assess how the disease is progressing.

Contact Tracing

In March 2020, a doctor who was working at a primary care facility run by the government of Delhi tested positive.[11] The doctor had attended to a patient who had returned from abroad. While the sample for the COVID-19 test for that patient was sent, the report was available only after six days and the patient was found positive. By then the doctor had already attended to nearly 900 patients. The samples of the doctor and his family were collected. People who had visited the clinic for consultation were contacted and asked to be

---

[11] Available at https://www.indiatoday.in/mail-today/story/coronavirus-in-india-900-quarantined-after-doctor-tests-positive-in-delhi-1660176-2020-03-27.

in home quarantine. Subsequently, the doctor, his wife and daughter were tested positive.

In the days to follow, the contact tracing exercise was done meticulously (described in Box 3.1 earlier). As phone numbers were not always available, many a time frontline health workers, wearing PPE, would have to visit the communities and trace the identified individuals. In certain densely populated areas, such as slums, it was a challenging task. More so, when people were not cooperative and even attacked the health workers.[12] However, for every confirmed case, nearly ten to fifty contacts were traced. The frontline health workers such as ASHAs or AWWs and others played a crucial role in this process.

Isolation and Quarantine

Early on, isolation was identified as an important tool to minimize the spread of the disease and a number of states had started setting up isolation facilities. In the beginning, isolation (for those who tested positive for COVID-19) was exclusively at a designated government facility (termed 'institutional isolation'). A few states had allowed health workers to be in home isolation as well. Setting up or strengthening existing isolation wards for COVID-19 cases in district hospitals was one of the first steps taken.

Quarantine is for healthy people but with travel or contact history. People waiting for their test results were usually

---

[12] Available at https://www.newindianexpress.com/nation/2020/apr/03/health-workers-under-attack-2125058.html

allowed to self-quarantine in their homes. However, if this was not possible, institutional quarantine was recommended. In the initial stages of the pandemic, the focus was on setting up institutional quarantine facilities. Vacant government buildings and flats were converted to quarantine facilities. Innovative approaches included the use of school premises, such as the Kendriya Vidyalaya (KV) and Jawahar Navodaya Vidyalaya (JNV), to create quarantine centres.[13]

Treat

Pandemics are best fought by public health and preventive and promotive strategies, such as test, trace and isolate (described earlier) and by breaking the chain of transmission. However, that is not always possible and when people get infected, we need to have treatment services ready. In COVID-19, all of the confirmed cases required consultation with health services and a proportion needed hospital-based medical management. Specific types of facilities and beds were needed and created for mild, moderate and severe patients (see Box 4.2).

---

[13] Available at https://www.hindustantimes.com/education/nearly-100-kvs-jnvs-turn-into-quarantine-health-facilities-to-fight-coronavirus/story-6qquPk4GomtCNklZD6BeGL.html.

Box 4.2 Types of COVID-19 Facilities and Provision of Beds in India

There are three main types of health facilities that have been developed/set up in India, for the treatment of COVID-19 cases:

- **Level 1: COVID Care Centres (CCC) for mild cases:** These are mainly to ensure isolation. Most of the patients here do not need any medical intervention.
- **Level 2: COVID Health Centre (CHC) for moderate cases:** Here a more watchful care is provided. These facilities have provision of beds with oxygen supply.
- **Level 3: Dedicated COVID Hospitals (DCH) for serious and critical cases:** These are equipped with ICU beds and ventilators.

Usually, every facility was created in a way that it catered to a specific stage of the disease; however, many of these designated facilities had a smaller number of beds to tackle the next level of the disease. This was done to ensure continuity of care when a patient becomes serious and needs more monitoring and support. In this way, no time is lost in providing the required type of care.

Getting the Health System Ready

The second objective of the lockdown was getting the health system ready for an effective pandemic response. The tools already identified to stop the spread of the virus could be effectively implemented by having a strengthened health system.[14] Two specific examples of how the administrative response was mounted through inter-ministerial and multi-sectoral participation, as well as through inter-sectoral participation within the ministry of health agencies, are summarized in Box 4.3. An indicative list of interventions carried out for the bolstering of health systems during this period are listed in Box 4.4.

Box 4.3: Governance Mechanisms and Team Approach

Inter-ministerial and Multi-Sectoral Participation and Response

The states have decision-making powers on matters of health and health services. However, this was a pandemic

---

[14] In chapters 9 and 10, we discuss how the strengthening of the health system is far broader and more comprehensive, though in popular narratives, it has been discussed in a simplistic sense of increasing hospital beds and ICUs alone.

and it needed a coordinated response. The response was coordinated at the highest level. It was led by the prime minister at the Union level and the chief ministers of the Indian states. India is a federal country where health is a subject assigned to the states. One of the earliest high-level committees was the Group of Ministers (GoM) formed in the first week of February 2020.[15] This included the cabinet ministers for union Ministry of Health and Family Welfare the MoHFW, civil aviation and external affairs, among others. Legal measures were also taken.

The response to health emergencies, epidemics and disasters are a part of the Concurrent List, as per the constitution of India.[16] The Disaster Management Act, 2005, and the Epidemic Diseases Act, 1897, were brought in to force. These provided the opportunity for a coordinated response to the pandemic.

---

[15] Available at https://www.outlookindia.com/newsscroll/group-of-ministers-formed-for-coronavirus/1725406.

[16] In the Constitution of India, the responsibilities between the Union and states have been distributed. These have been grouped under three lists. The Union List and State List have those areas which are the exclusive responsibility of the Union and state governments. For example, defence is in the Union list and health in the state list. The third, the Concurrent List has those subjects where a decision can be made by both Union and state governments. However, in this list, the decision or law of the Union government supersedes the state law.

On policies and at the administrative level, the ministry of home affairs constituted eleven empowered groups to deliberate on various aspects of the response to the pandemic. These were chaired by Secretaries to the Government of India who were in charge of various departments or a higher level of officials who represented other relevant ministries. These empowered groups were given the authority to identify problem areas and provide effective solutions. The responsibilities included delineating policies, formulating plans, strategizing operations and taking all the necessary steps for effective and time-bound implementation of these policies/ strategies and decisions.

Inter-disciplinary Engagement between Health Agencies

On the technical aspects of dealing with the pandemic, the MoHFW and allied divisions, departments and units, including DGHS, NCDC and the Indian Council of Medical Research (ICMR), were working round the clock. The JMG in DGHS under the MoHFW was working regularly on various aspects of planning. A Strategic Health Operations Centre (SHOC) room (colloquially called the 'War' room) was set up in Nirman Bhawan, New Delhi. ICMR had set up a national public health task force and several technical sub-committees to guide the response. The NCDC was coordinating through its field centres across the country for the various surveillance activities.

Team Approach at Union and State Levels and within Health Facilities

The Union government regularly formed and dispatched public health teams to various states and districts, which coordinated with the states and contributed to help them review and redesign the response. Experts affiliated with various institutions were members of these teams.

The team approach in the delivery of health services at the facility levels was never more visible (and needed) as doctors, nurses, ward boys and attendants in hospitals came together to play their roles. Outside the hospitals and in the communities, frontline health workers, the police (booth-level officers), schoolteachers and sanitation workers—everyone worked hard in their respective roles to ensure that the infection did not spread at a pace that would overwhelm the hospitals.

Box 4.4 Getting Health Systems Ready
(Indicative list)

Leadership, Policy Interventions and Regulation

- The prime minister at the national level and chief ministers at the state level steered the response.

- The GoM met regularly to coordinate pandemic response at the national level.
- Teleconsultation guidelines approved by the Board of Governors (BoG) of the then Medical Council of India (MCI).
- Home delivery and online sale of medicines were allowed
- Many approvals from the Central Drugs Standard Control Organisation (CDSCO) were granted in an expedited manner, for instance, for RT-PCR test kits and viral extraction kits.
- Any attack on health workers was made a non-bailable offence.
- A health insurance cover of Rs 50 lakh for health professionals was announced under the Pradhan Mantri Garib Kalyan Yojana.

Financial Allocation

- A sum of Rs 15,000 crore was allocated by the Union government, specifically for the pandemic.
- The PM CARES fund was initiated.

Testing Kits and Other Measures

- Laboratory capacity for COVID-19 testing was rapidly expanded.
- Increased the production capacity of viral transport medium for testing kits.

- India adopted the approach of 'pooled testing'[17] to reduce cost and efficiently use the available resources.
- The indigenously developed TrueNAT and CBNAAT[18] machines were used to increase COVID-19 testing.
- The testing laboratories across the country were strengthened, specially in the remotest parts of the country.
- For the first time, many of the districts purchased oxygen concentrators.
- The Defence Research Development Organisation (DRDO) set up oxygen concentrator plants in far-flung hospitals.
- The manufacturing capacity for ventilators was increased from 3000 a month in February to 33,000 a month in May 2020.

Health Workforce

- The capacity-building of the staff in various government facilities had begun.
- The government requested all states to fill the vacancies for epidemiologists and the district surveillance officers

---

[17] Available at https://www.livemint.com/news/india/pooling-can-help-india-optimize-its-testing-strategy-11587578644506.html.
[18] TrueNat is a molecular test that can diagnose tuberculosis (TB). CBNAAT stands for cartridge-based nucleic acid amplification test and is extensively used to test TB in India.

immediately. A proposal was mooted to recruit nearly 300 epidemiologists and public health specialists in the Union ministry of health and related institutions.

- The government of Delhi announced an insurance of Rs 1 crore for any individual who would die on corona duty.
- The services of schoolteachers, booth-level officers and employees of other departments were sought, to address the shortage of frontline workers.
- In a few states, the final-year nursing and medical students were roped in for COVID-19 duties.

Health Infrastructure and Services

- By the time lockdown ended, nearly 3 lakh COVID-specific hospital beds were ready. A total of 7 lakh isolation beds were made available for mild cases.[19]
- CCCs were set up in schools and colleges that had been converted into isolation and quarantine facilities.
- State roadways buses were converted into mobile clinics to ensure adequate availability of medical services.
- CCCs were created in residential areas by making use of the vacant flats.

---

[19] Available at https://www.pib.gov.in/PressReleseDetailm.aspx?PRID=1629672.

Other Interventions

- RCCE interventions were implemented across the country.
- A few states empowered the elected local self-government (Panchayati Raj institutions and panchayat members) to conduct house-to-house screening and granted them other decision-making powers for the COVID-19 response.

Challenges and Learnings

During the pandemic there were numerous reports on the challenges and struggle of both people and health staff in accessing and delivering services, respectively. Most of these arguably reflected amplified versions of existing challenges of the health system. Some of these have been tackled partially for COVID-19; however, it is important that these are documented and then addressed for the long term as well. A few challenges that emerged have been discussed here.

The health services were temporarily disrupted. Many government and private health facilities were closed. The non-COVID-19 essential health services were reduced in a majority of government and private-sector facilities. The Government of India had issued an advisory on the continuity of essential health services, yet there was a noticeable reduction in provision of health services at the field level. The testing facilities were limited and there were reports of some laboratories charging excessively for the tests, even though the government had put a price cap on the RT-PCR test. The basic and advanced life-support ambulances were in short supply.

There was a lot of discourse on ventilators in hospitals in India. In addition to the shortage of ventilators in general, it emerged that most district hospitals had just one or a few ventilators, the majority of which were non-functional. The specialists required to keep the ventilators running on a regular basis were not available in the districts. In most of the remote districts, even ambulance services were augmented by the hiring of private vehicles, drivers and other ancillary staff. Though COVID-19-specific health facilities were getting ready, making those functional was the real challenge.

Private healthcare facilities remained largely underutilized or closed. However, when these started to open, in a majority of these facilities the consultation fees as well as the charges for rooms and other services were hiked by 40 to 50 per cent. The cost of treatment for COVID-19 patients was very high and ranged from Rs 3 to 16 lakh per patient with the minimum payment usually starting at three lakh.[20]

In the initial stage, the people who tested positive for COVID-19 and their family members were discriminated against and stigmatized. There were reports that people stopped interacting with health workers, and many were

---

[20] M. Kaunain Sherif, 'Rs 3-16 Lakh: In COVID bills, drug cost, PPE are main unknowns', 28 May 2020. Available at https://indianexpress.com/article/india/rs-3-16-lakh-in-COVID-bills-drug-cost-ppe-are-main-unknowns/.

socially boycotted. People stopped talking to them and their family members and even abused them. The health workers assigned with the task of contact tracing were attacked in a number of cities.

The pandemic has once more shown that health and disease affect society and economy alike. The stoppage of public transport, including the sealing of district and state borders, caused a lot of inconvenience to many people. Work in factories and other settings stopped. The situation affected nearly everyone; however, informal sector workers including migrants were the most affected. Their earnings were drastically reduced, compounded by the fact that during the initial days, even accessing essential services was a challenge. As transport facilities shut down, many migrants started walking back home, which was often hundreds of kilometres away. The pandemic had a different face in the form of migrants on the road. Mental health issues were also increasingly being observed and reported during the pandemic period. This was all a reflection of the human impact of a health crisis. This is a subject which needs to be studied. In a few cases solutions emerged but not immediately.

How Did India Fare During the Lockdown?

Any assessment of the country's performance during the lockdown needs to focus on the stated objectives of slowing the spread of the virus and strengthening health systems. By the end of May 2020, numbers of COVID-19 cases in India were not as high as the model-based estimates had projected on 24 March 2020. However, inferring that the gap between projected and actual cases reflects the impact of the lockdown would also be too simplistic an analysis. To assess the impact of the lockdown on halting the virus, a number of modelling-based analyses were done by various agencies. Most of these models estimated that in India 15 to 30 lakh COVID-19 cases and 37,000 to 78,000 deaths had been averted by 15 May 2020.[21] Though the estimates were variable, there was broader agreement that the virus spread had been slowed down.

When the Lockdown Was about to Be Lifted

St Xaviers College, Mumbai, is among India's top colleges. In the last week of May 2020, the front pages of newspapers were splattered with images of the iconic college hall of St Xavier College. The hall had been converted into a quarantine centre and beds were put in the area. Mehboob Studio in Mumbai (famous for iconic movies and a landmark in the city) and the J.J. School of Applied Art were among other private facilities which were converted to COVID-Care Centres. People would have never dreamt of these spaces being used for such a purpose. However, that was the case in May 2020.

The city of Mumbai was converting many large grounds and complexes to either quarantine centres or COVID-19 facilities. Delhi was looking at marriage halls, community halls and banquet halls to convert them to COVID-19 centres.

---

[21] Available at https://indianexpress.com/article/explained/how-many-deaths-prevented-6441365/.

Across the country, schools, colleges and training centres were being used, secured and converted to respond to the pandemic. In Delhi, the government had started the process to rope in private hotels for COVID-19 treatment services, by putting in the beds and as admission centres.[22] Five leading private hotels were linked to five private hospitals. This was being done in anticipation of the surge in cases that was likely to happen once the lockdown was lifted.

The state of Karnataka was completing a household survey, where they collected information on high-risk people.[23] The state government was discussing the importance and relevance of a comprehensive public health database for effective and timely interventions in the field of health and medical care.

Across India, other cities were focusing on setting up more quarantine centres and isolation facilities of various types.

At the end of May 2020, in Delhi, a few medical directors and heads of leading medical institutions and a deputy commissioner of police tested positive for COVID-19. There had been many cases of health workers who had been infected, a few had died and many were under home quarantine.[24]

---

[22] Available at https://www.newindianexpress.com/cities/delhi/2020/may/30/delhi-government-designates-five-hotels-to-increase-capacity-of-COVID-19-dedicated-hospitals--2149967.html.

[23] Available at https://www.deccanherald.com/state/karnataka-districts/karnataka-government-survey-puts-5887-lakh-households-in-COVID-19-risk-category-845842.html.

[24] Available at https://indianexpress.com/article/cities/delhi/delhi-coronavirus-health-workers-doctors-aiims-gtb-hospital-6434331/.

The sixty-eight days of lockdown were nearly over. Experts were deliberating on the best way to achieve a balance of economic and social activities to prevent the spread of the virus. Protecting the frontline workers was identified as a priority in order to keep the health services running.

Alongside, the stories of the trials and tribulations of the people seeking non-COVID-19 essential health services emerged. In Raipur, Chhattisgarh, a pregnant woman faced a lot of challenges when she was about to deliver her baby in the first week of the lockdown. The struggle and concern about COVID-19 was so overwhelming for the couple that when the mother delivered twins, the couple reportedly named their children Corona and Covid (which they later changed).

The nationwide lockdown was lifted on 31 May 2020 at 11:59 pm. Unlock 1 had begun.

What Did Everyone Learn during This Period?

- **Health is much more than medical care or treating only sick people.** The importance of public health services in preventing diseases, protecting people and maintaining health was being recognized. Even beyond the pandemic, if preventive and promotive measures are implemented well, these can reverse the ongoing silent pandemics of non-communicable diseases including diabetes and hypertension.

- **Communities have a role in keeping society healthy and protected.** People adopted and adhered to non-pharmacological interventions of using face masks, handwashing and physical distancing and that's how the pandemic was confronted. The need for hospital services can be reduced with effective implementation of preventive and promotive protocols by the government and their adherence by the people.

- **Frontline health workers, including community health workers, are the foundation of health services.** Be it contact tracing, running isolation facilities, COVID-19 testing services, or delivering services at the hospitals, a wide range of community-level workers and health staff were fighting at the frontline to halt the virus and the pandemic.

- **Well-functioning health systems require sustained high-level leadership at all levels.** It was sustained and top-level political leadership which steered the response to the pandemic. It needs to be sustained in the period beyond the pandemic as well. Stronger health systems are possible only through the highest level of leadership.

- **There are shortages of supplies and equipment in government facilities.** The shortage of PPE and ventilators identified during the early stage of the pandemic can be considered as tracer indicators of the shortage of some of the inputs and supplies (medicines and testing services), which are essential to deliver health services.[25]

- **Many equate medical care with healthcare, but the two are not the same.** The excessive projection and attention on hospital beds and ventilators is also an indication that it is often medical care that is equated with healthcare. In reality, public health and social measures are equally useful in a pandemic response as well as in routine services.

- **Health systems means much more than hospitals.** During the pandemic, there have been a lot of references to the strengthening of health systems, which was often discussed in the narrow sense of increasing COVID-19 testing capacity, as well as provision of hospital beds (with the focus being on ICU and ventilators). However, health systems strengthening is a much broader concept. (Discussed in Chapter 9.)

- **Sometimes, health systems and institutions need to be challenged to perform optimally.** During the pandemic, several health institutes and facilities were stretched. It was this challenge which nudged and geared these facilities to get prepared for an adequate response.

---

[25] Available at https://main.mohfw.gov.in/sites/default/files/71275472221489753307.pdf.

5

The Unlock: Balancing Safety and Economy

Dharavi is a slum in Mumbai that houses nearly a million people, most of them migrant workers, in 2.5-square-kilometre area. In single hutment of 8x10 feet, around ten people stay. There are multistorey hutments. There are common toilets and bathing facilities. Daily-wage earners comprise 70 per cent of the population and 80 per cent use community toilets.[1] Community taps and tankers are their main source of water. Being an extremely valuable resource, water was unlikely to be used for frequent handwashing. Overcrowding made social distancing impossible. Due to all this, experts had reason to fear that if COVID-19 cases emerged in Dharavi, things would go out of hand quickly. Among the measures that could be taken, the wearing of masks

---

[1] Available at https://theprint.in/opinion/dharavis-unexpected-COVID-success-story-has-lessons-for-delhi-other-crowded-cities/441726/.

seemed to be an idea that would be acceptable to the people, but it would probably not be enough. Masks also need to be purchased. The price may be low but it could be significant from the perspective of someone living in Dharavi. Choices can sometimes be very challenging: buy a mask or get a meal?

Mumbai, a metropolitan city and the financial capital of India, with an estimated population of around 20 million, had been reporting the maximum number of cases in India, since the pandemic began in India. Alarm bells had started to ring as soon as the first COVID-19 case and death from Dharavi was reported on 1 April 2020.

The first standard response of the authorities was to declare Dharavi a containment zone. Barricades were put up all around the locality. Corporation workers dressed in full PPE coveralls were sent to the slum to conduct a house-to-house survey, with the aim of contact tracing. This approach received little response. Most teams of health workers were treated with hostility. Most of the slum-dwellers did not reveal the actual number of people residing in the hutment. Once they learnt that the health workers had been sent by the municipal corporation, they did not even reveal if they had any symptoms. This attitude was not specific to Mumbai. Slum dwellers in urban areas generally harbour a deep mistrust towards the governments and corporations, as they are very often considered illegal occupants. Thus, whenever these surveys were being conducted, the responses were protracted and the attitude uncooperative. They feared that later on the government might use that information to evict them. Declaring the area a containment zone and then sending healthcare workers for surveys only served to increase their suspicion. After screening nearly 5 per cent of the target population, the corporation changed its strategy. It decided to adapt itself locally to make the exercise people-friendly.

The containment approach was supplemented by easy access to COVID-19 testing services, which were offered free of cost to all those who had symptoms and were suspected cases. The government also made an additional provision of continued supply of essential goods. Water supply was increased and other services such as sanitation were enhanced. The community now felt that this was for their own good.

A few fever clinics were set up in the locality. Since there was a shortage of government staff and doctors, the services of private-sector doctors, who were already serving in these localities, were used. The inhabitants were used to visiting these private doctors and had faith in them. A mass communication campaign was conducted in the area to sensitize people to come to the fever clinics and get check-ups done. The private doctors were paid by the government and the services were free for the people. Visits to these clinics were voluntary, and people started to approach them. More than half of the total population came forward for screening in the first few weeks. Many of them visited repeatedly at an early stage of their symptoms.

After consulting technical experts, the strategy for contact tracing was also modified. Earlier, around fifteen contacts of every case were being traced. In the revised strategy, a pragmatic approach was adopted whereby only those people who had been sharing the room with the patient and using the same community toilets were considered contacts.

The local authorities had set up quarantine facilities in schools, hotels and community halls. Anyone who was identified as a contact of a patient was given the option of being quarantined in these institutional facilities. Once admitted, food and basic necessities were supplied. Once word spread about the cleanliness and services at the quarantine centres, people volunteered to be admitted to these at the earliest sign of risk. If any of them tested positive, they were quickly shifted to the designated isolation facilities. There were reports that several patients who came to the quarantine centres showed no symptoms, but their physical and mental health deteriorated due to stress and panic.

Isolation facilities and CCCs were set up locally. Nine out of every ten patients were treated in these local centres. This was reassuring for everyone. At the centres, people received round-the-clock care and medical supervision at no cost. For treatment of severe cases and for critical care, the authorities took over the private hospitals in that area.

Cases were on the rise for the first few weeks. However, once the strategies were stabilized, the spread slowed down.

It was a success story arrived at through adaptation, in a people-friendly way, of known public-health interventions for pandemic control. Dharavi's response to the COVID-19 pandemic is an example of what people, public health and government authorities can achieve with appropriate interventions and community participation.

By the time the lockdown in the country was being lifted, Dharavi had already reversed the trend.

The Lockdown and the States: A Tale of Differences

Everyone in India wished for a flattened pandemic curve; however, the virus seemed to have a different plan. During the lockdown, there were a few insights and learnings. First, it became evident that the approach of test, detect, trace, isolate and treat was the right strategy. Second, the lockdown allowed time for capacity building of health staff and for improving infrastructure. Third, the learnings from other countries in pandemic response helped to develop strategies here. Fourth, there was a better understanding of who is likely to develop serious symptoms of the disease: those older than sixty years, and people with underlying health conditions or comorbidities. This information was useful to focus on interventions to prevent deaths in these high-risk subgroups. Fifth, it was in the lockdown period that we learnt that around one in every five confirmed cases would need oxygen support. Sixth, we also learnt that severe symptoms of the disease are witnessed in only 3 to 5 per cent of the laboratory-confirmed cases, and these were the people who would require critical care, that is, ICU and/or ventilator support. Seventh, the experts identified some of the existing drugs and therapies with the potential to save life (more on this in chapter 7).

Other than Dharavi in Mumbai, of the all the states and districts termed as 'model' and labelled as a success story, at a state level, Kerala stood out. Of the total of 191,000 cases reported from India till 31 May 2020, nearly 1200 cases were from Kerala.[2] It had implemented an extensive testing strategy and effective contact tracing. The strategies were guided by

---

[2]   Available at COVID19India.org; data accessed for 31 May 2020.

experts and regularly updated. These were coupled with good treatment. Unlike a few other states, even the return of migrant workers did not disturb the balance and the state was doing really well on containing the virus. Many factors were attributed to its success: (a) a strong government-funded primary healthcare system developed over the last six decades; (b) a state government that had experience in handling crises, for instance, the Nipah outbreaks of 2018 and 2019 and the Kerala floods; (c) active community participation and (d) the use of technology for contact tracing.

Another characteristic of the pandemic in the initial few months was that most cases were from urban settings. A majority of cases were from Mumbai, Delhi, Ahmedabad, Surat, Jaipur, Indore and Pune. On a positive note, one city was apparently doing far better than others: Bengaluru. In fact, it was doing better in comparison to the other districts within the state of Karnataka as well. In early June, Bengaluru was touted as a model for pandemic response.[3] A stringent lockdown, household surveys and strict adherence to institutional isolation for returning migrants were credited for the city's success until then.

The Press Conference in Delhi

On the evening of 9 June, the deputy chief minister of Delhi had just stepped out after attending a meeting of the Delhi

---

[3] Available at https://www.newindianexpress.com/states/ karnataka/2020/jun/15/in-coronavirus-vs-karnataka-the-state- shines-against-all-odds-2156665.html.

Disaster Management Authority. He addressed the media and announced that in the coming weeks, as per projections and estimates, COVID-19 cases were going to rise rapidly in Delhi. The projections were that there would be 5.5 lakh cases and the need for 80,000 COVID-19 beds by 31 July 2020.[4] The state had nearly 15,000 COVID-19 beds combining both the public and private sectors. The news made its way to the front pages of newspapers across India. The chief minister of Delhi termed the need for arranging 100,000 beds as 'unprecedented and a huge challenge'.

As epidemiological understanding evolved, it was clear that a majority, nearly 80 per cent, of the COVID-19 cases had mild symptoms. These patients with mild symptoms were recovering without significant medical intervention. Keeping these mild patients in hospitals would reduce the availability of beds, which were required for moderate and serious patients who needed direct medical observation. Though initially proposed only for health staff, starting early May 2020, the state of Delhi was already implementing the home isolation strategy for the general public as well (see Box 5.1). The strategy seemed to have worked and it reduced the burden on the healthcare sector. Around 10 June 2020, nearly one-third of all the active COVID-19 cases in Delhi were under home isolation. Yet, there was an impending shortage of hospital beds for moderate and serious cases. Something needed to be done.

---

[4] Available at https://www.business-standard.com/article/current-affairs/delhi-COVID-19-cases-may-mount-to-550-000-in-by-july-31-manish-sisodia-120060900650_1.html.

Box 5.1 The Home Isolation Strategy in Delhi

Initially, every COVID-19 patient who had tested positive was supposed to be admitted to a designated facility. However, the health staff who tested positive were allowed to be isolated at home. It was soon recognized that many of the patients experiencing mild symptoms were not keen to be admitted to the health facilities. Admission in COVID-care centres meant being disconnected from their family members. It was a cause of worry for the families as well. The government of Delhi allowed home isolation on certain conditions such as availability of a separate room with an attached bathroom, and so on. Before the home isolation would begin, a health team would reach the house and assess whether it met the criteria and it would disinfect all the areas and rooms in the house. A hired agency would conduct telephonic follow-ups twice a day.

This approach became immensely popular with the people. More and more people were willing to get tested. In the weeks that followed, by July 2020, it became a key strategy for effective management of mild COVID-19 cases. The patients in home isolation were handed over pulse oximeters to regularly measure their oxygen saturation levels. The devices were to be returned to the government once the isolation period was over. At various points of time, half or more of the active COVID-19 cases were under home isolation in Delhi. A number of other states adopted this strategy in the period to follow.

A Coordinated Response to an Impending Crisis

The disease modelling–based projections have limitations in general. Yet, uncertainties notwithstanding, when such projections are made, to not do anything is never an option. The operational question was how to prepare for such an eventuality? How to arrange for so many beds? The search for stadia, banquet halls and hotels in order to convert them to makeshift care centres and hospitals started. The government issued orders to the private hospitals to increase the number of beds for COVID-19 patients. A few private hospitals were directed to become dedicated COVID-19 facilities.

In the days to follow, as the number of cases soared, the available beds were rapidly being occupied by the COVID-19 cases. Most of the hospitals in the private sector were running at nearly full capacity with regard to COVID-19 patients. The principle of economics pertaining to supply and demand is of great relevance in the health sector as well. The rates of hospital beds and cost of treatment skyrocketed, and many private hospitals were reportedly charging from Rs 50,000 to Rs 70,000 per night for beds in the ICUs.[5] Health services have nearly always been unaffordable for the poor and marginalized, they were now beyond the reach of even the affluent citizens.

---

[5] 'Coronavirus: SC directs Centre to cap cost of treatment at private hospitals as cases cross 9 lakh', Scroll.in, 14 July 2020. Available at https://scroll.in/latest/967415/coronavirus-there-will-be-no-return-to-old-normal-for-the-foreseeable-future-warns-who.

The public acknowledgement of the need for more hospital beds in Delhi gave rise to a lot of speculation. Newspaper headlines started speculating if Delhi was going to be India's New York City (the city of New York was among the worst affected in the pandemic in the USA).

There were talks of another lockdown in the metropolis as the only solution, which were later dispelled by state government.[6] If the pandemic could not be contained in a city such as Delhi, which had one of the best public and private sector healthcare facilities, was the seat of power of the Union government, and home to policymakers and experts who were advising the rest of the country, it was bound to set tongues wagging about India's preparedness for and response to a health crisis.

The fear of such an outcome perhaps encouraged several agencies to get into action. Even within the state of Delhi multiple agencies deliver health services with limited coordination. A number of facilities are also run by the Union Government of India, a few by four corporations and many more by various autonomous agencies. The state government led by the chief minister, the lieutenant governor of Delhi, the Union home ministry, and the municipal corporations all started to coordinate with each other. A series of meetings at the highest levels of these agencies were convened and leading experts were roped in. A joint action plan was drafted to combat the emerging situation and every stakeholder was expected to do their bit (Box 5.2).

---

[6] Available at https://indianexpress.com/article/cities/delhi/delhi-lockdown-COVID-19-6456246/.

Box 5.2 Joint Strategies and Actions Taken to Respond to the COVID-19 Surge in Delhi, June 2020

- Containment zones redefined and reclassified; interventions strengthened.
- Testing services accelerated and sustained thereafter.
- House-to-house surveys to be regularly conducted in containment zones and other identified areas.
- Contact tracing improved and additional human resources deployed.
- Isolation beds increased by setting up dedicated facilities in banquet halls, stadia and on the grounds.
- For expanding treatment services, ICU beds and beds with oxygen support in government facilities were ramped up.

Within a few days, specific interventions to implement the strategies were initiated. One major hospital run by the municipal corporation was converted to a COVID-19 only facility. To increase the testing rate and overcome the shortage of RT-PCR testing capacity, the use of RAT kits in containment zones was approved.

Getting ready with that many beds was probably the biggest challenge. A plan was announced to set up a 10,000-bed CCC. Even rail coaches were used as isolation wards. The work started and completed on all these fronts including setting up 10,000-bed CCC in Chhatarpur.

There were several other challenges that remained to be addressed. An expert panel was set up to review the cost of COVID-19 beds in hospitals. The panel came up with a new cost structure for private hospitals (government hospitals provide all services for free), which was enforced in Delhi and later a few other states also adopted a similar approach of price capping on services. The price of COVID-19 testing in private laboratories was capped at Rs 2400 (again, it was free in the government-run labs).

Around 10 June 2020 nearly 1350 new COVID-19 cases started to be reported per day in Delhi. The number of daily new cases increased to 3900 on 23 June 2020.[7] The number of cumulative cases had increased from 31,000 to 66,000 in two weeks. All eyes were now on Delhi.

The Challenges in Delhi's COVID-19 response

It was not without challenges and there were hurdles in expanding testing services. The hotels where rooms or conference halls were supposed to be made available as extended hospital beds/wards went to the court against the government order. The COVID-19 testing strategies changed regularly, which at times created confusion. The service of the agency supporting the tele-follow-up for patients in home isolation was terminated on procedural grounds. For a short period, the home isolation guidelines were modified, and every patient was asked to be admitted to institutional isolation for the initial five days.

---

[7]   Available at COVID19India.org.

There were days when things were chaotic in the cities, and it was the same for all cities. From many parts of the country there were reports of serious non-COVID-19 patients being denied services at both government and private facilities.

Technology is a helpful friend but not always. A mobile-based application was created to track the availability of COVID-19 beds in hospitals in Delhi. However, it was only partially useful. The data was not being updated in real time and the app had limited utility. It underscored the importance of balance and coordination between the reliance on technology and human interface.

Isolation centres were created in various empty flats in the outskirts of Delhi. However, the distance and services left patients unhappy. The residents in the area also complained about isolation centres being set up closer to their homes. They were afraid of the centre bringing infection to their locality or residential areas. Moreover, the location of the isolation centres in the outskirts meant that ambulances took a long time to ferry patients.

A few reports had also emerged alleging that dead bodies were not being removed in a timely manner from the wards.

Strengthening the health system comes with its own set of challenges. A weak health system cannot be improved drastically in such a short span of time. The remedy lies in government investment in health services at a time when there is no emergency.

On 31 July 2020, Delhi did not report 550,000 cases, nor did it need 80,000 hospital beds. In fact, till that day,

Delhi reported a cumulative total of 136,000 cases, 3960 deaths, and had 10,700 active cases.[8] The projections made by the technical experts and the government had been incorrect. However, one of the measures of effectiveness of public health interventions is reducing adverse outcomes. Arguably, in many ways, the impact of interventions from 10 June to 31 July 2020 was visible in the difference in the projected number of cases and the actual case and death count.

How can Delhi's response be summarized? In an interview with a leading newspaper, the chief minister of Delhi described three principles of teamwork: acknowledging constructive criticism, fixing what is wrong and not giving up as the government no matter how bad the situation.

Why Learnings from Delhi Are Relevant for the Entire country?

This book has documented Delhi's fight against COVID-19 in greater detail than that of any other state in India. There are multiple reasons for this. Delhi was the first state where such a risk was explicitly recognized by the government and actions were proposed and initiated. The state also presented one of the highest levels of challenges faced at the planning unit level. If the pandemic could be tackled in a city with a population of two crore or twenty million, it gives hope that through concerted actions, the pandemic can be managed in any of the metro cities and also at the district level

---

[8]   Available at www.COVID19India.org; accessed for 31 July 2020.

in India, which have far smaller populations (but also limited resources). The key lessons from Delhi's response to the pandemic are summarized in Box 5.3.

Box 5.3 Key Learnings from Delhi's Fight against COVID-19

- The approach of containment, test, trace, isolate and treat has been proven effective. All that is needed is locally adapted and accelerated implementation.
- We cannot drop our guard till the pandemic is fully over; interventions at all levels (individual, public health and medical care) need to be continued.
- People's participation in COVID-19-appropriate behaviour and effective implementation of non-pharmacological interventions are essential.
- For effective response in health emergencies, both public and private sectors need to pool their resources. Everyone needs to be engaged. Legal and other approaches need to be sought, if necessary.
- Transparent communication about the disease and government interventions is a must.
- An explicit recognition of the problem by the government can open channels for a coordinated response.
- Teamwork is essential for an effective response: Government leadership as well as multi-sectoral participation is crucial.

COVID-19 in Rural India: An Early Insight

In rural India, Bihar, a largely rural state with relatively weak health infrastructure, felt the heat first. In the month of July, the cases in Bihar increased fivefold.[9] Cases were being reported from nearly all the districts. The challenges which people faced in accessing routine healthcare services had multiplied. The shortage of hospital beds (especially for COVID-19) as well as beds with oxygen support was identified as a major challenge. There were barely a few functional ventilators even in medical colleges. The shortage of healthcare staff and vacancies in government facilities were felt acutely. Newspapers were once again filled with stories of the trials and tribulations of the patients seeking care.

This was not the story of Bihar alone. Over a period of time, the situation and pattern of cases in rural India followed a similar trajectory. More cases emerged in Madhya Pradesh, Chhattisgarh, Rajasthan, Gujarat and many other states. Essentially, not a single state was spared, though the extent remained variable; in some parts of the country, such as the north-east, cases emerged a little later.

The Tables Turned: From Success to Challenges

If any state was thought to have won the war against COVID-19, every such inference was proven premature. The first 1000 cases in Kerala had been reported over nearly

---

[9] Available at https://www.deccanherald.com/national/east-and-northeast/bihar-COVID-19-tally-breaches-50000-mark-with-highest-one-day-spike-of-2986-cases-868067.html.

four months. However, in mid-July, in a single day, the state reported nearly 800 cases. By early September 2020, the state had more active cases than a city like Delhi. It had taken four and a half months for the state to report its first 10,000 cases. However, almost the same number of cases was reported in a single day in October 2020. This situation clearly highlights how unpredictable pandemics are. Yet, Kerala's experience also highlights the importance of a strong foundation for a good start in health emergencies such as outbreaks and epidemics. The healthcare system in Kerala helped in ensuring that medical services were not overwhelmed and people did not panic. However, as pandemics and diseases evolve, the strategies to tackle them also need to evolve. Whenever that did not happen, it resulted a new localized surge.

Similarly, until early June the state of Karnataka and Bengaluru city were being considered as model in terms of their response to COVID-19. Within three weeks in the month of June, Bengaluru became the epicentre of COVID-19 in Karnataka. Between 1 to 30 June, the number of cases in Bengaluru increased from 385 to 4500. Once the number went up, the city adopted its own set of trial-and-error approach response. As with other cities, along with the spike in positive cases, there was a sudden shortage of hospital beds, staff and ICUs. There were also reports of a patient being refused admission by eighteen hospitals before he died.[10] Understandably, the administration issued a notice to all these facilities.

---

[10] Available at https://theprint.in/india/bengaluru-man-dies-after-18-hospitals-deny-admission-govt-issues-notice-to-9/452614/.

Delhi in September 2020: A Different Storyline

In September 2020, the number of COVID-19 cases once again increased in Delhi. However, by this time the situation was completely different. There was no panic. Hospitals were not overwhelmed. A system was in place. The home isolation approach ensured that large temporary COVID-19 centres were not required. Health workers were thus available to serve moderate and severe cases. The case fatality rates had come down.[11] The test, isolate and treat approach had been strengthened since June 2020. The state had already ramped up COVID-19 testing, which was now allowed without a prescription. The timings of state-run dispensaries and urban primary health centres (UPHCs) were extended to accommodate testing services. Testing centres were set up in the Interstate Bus Terminal (ISBT) and mohalla clinics were roped in to offer testing services as well.

Battling Social (and Societal) Biases

Dr Sanjay Gangurde was working at a district hospital in Nashik, Maharashtra, in a dedicated COVID-19 ward. In the initial days of the pandemic, when he would return home, the members of the housing society where he lived would welcome him with claps and hail him as a corona warrior. Sometime later, he tested positive for COVID-19 with mild symptoms, and he was advised to stay in isolation. However,

---

[11] Available at https://www.hindustantimes.com/india-news/india-s-COVID-toll-100-000/story-sNGsNLCA2MjbpMfjDdFEDI.html.

at that point, the members of the housing society passed a resolution to bar his entry into the society. When he returned home, he was not allowed to enter his building. He finally isolated himself along with his wife (who had also tested positive) in a room of the same hospital where he worked.[12]

The response to the pandemic was adversely affected by the prevailing social biases and stigma. A leading doctor in Delhi described how people in his locality nearly ostracized him when he was tested positive for COVID-19. When he was in isolation, the same group of people who had earlier sought his help boycotted him.[13]

There have been stories of doctors, nurses and other health staff being abused in the streets. They were asked to vacate their accommodation and were barred from entering their homes. People saw them as a potential source of infection. Those belonging to the north-eastern parts of India were abused with racist slurs and (wrongly) blamed for the spread of the disease.

These biases had always existed in our society, but they became more pronounced during the pandemic, risking the joint fight against COVID-19. Apparently, in the later months, reports of such cases emerged less frequently. However, it was clear that we as a society needed to fight

---

[12] Available at https://indianexpress.com/article/india/nashik-doctor-tests-positive-advised-home-isolation-but-neighbours-bar-his-entry-6399345/.

[13] Available at https://www.hindustantimes.com/analysis/i-had-COVID-19-and-society-decided-to-stigmatise-me/story-pwLgTsUbUycqrAqI9CAROL.html.

against these biases as much as we needed to fight the COVID-19 pandemic.

Mental Health Needs and Services: Another Revelation

Experts have always argued that the importance of mental health has not been sufficiently recognized in India and mental health services are insufficient. One of the reasons is that mental health needs are not considered at par with physical illnesses and have historically been stigmatized. In a 2017 study on the burden of mental health in India, it was estimated that there are nearly 200 million people suffering from some form of mental disorders in India.[14] During the pandemic, there was an increased need and demand for mental healthcare services in all parts of the country. A national-level mental healthcare helpline was set up. The healthcare staff and community members were stressed. Families were stressed due to the fears related to COVID-19 or the fear of loss of income. The challenges faced by people during the pandemic have highlighted the need for the urgent scaling up of mental healthcare services in India. We need not to wait for the pandemic to be over to address this. Something must be done now.

---

[14] 'The burden of mental disorders across the states of India: The Global Burden of Disease Study 1990–2017', *Lancet Psychiatry*, February 2020. Available at https://www.thelancet.com/journals/lanpsy/article/PIIS2215-0366(19)30475-4/fulltext.

There is a gross shortage of mental healthcare professionals in India. This holds true at every level and for nearly all subgroups of health staff. Much of these services are restricted to the district level.[15] Although India released a national mental health policy in 2014 and a legal mechanism in the form of the Mental Healthcare Act, 2017, it still has a long way to go towards bolstering mental healthcare services in the country.

Mental healthcare facilities need to be made accessible to all through primary healthcare services. While we need to have more specialist doctors and mental health counsellors, there is also an urgent need for community mental health workers.

Community Engagement and Participation

Dr Raj and Mabelle Arole are a famous doctor couple from the state of Maharashtra. Back in the 1970s, they returned from the USA after completing their higher studies in public health. They wanted to set up primary healthcare services in rural Maharashtra. Their idea was to involve the community in the process. They started meeting the community members and seeking their inputs on what type of health services they needed.

When they initially met the community members in various villages, the villagers were barely allowed to speak. In

---

[15] Available at https://www.thehindu.com/sci-tech/health/policy-and-issues/acute-shortage-of-mental-health-care-staff-in-india/article4305058.ece.

one of the cases, the village leader insisted that his voice was the only voice which mattered and his people would follow him. The doctors were not expecting this kind of response. Later, the doctor duo built a primary healthcare system in Jamkhed, Maharashtra, which became a model for the rest of the world for community participation in the delivery of health services. Nearly fifty years later, in an article in *BMJ Global Health*, a few public health experts analysed this approach and concluded: 'The most sustainable and effective partnerships are explicitly three way partnerships involving grassroots citizens, local political leaders and technical health experts.'[16]

This paper was published nearly a year before the COVID-19 pandemic. However, what actually worked was essentially a three-way partnership between elected political leaders, citizens and community members, and technical (public health and medical health) experts. Community participation in pandemic response is indispensable and cannot be overemphasized.

The success of face masks, social distancing and handwashing will be limited till most people adopt and adhere to these behaviours. COVID-19 testing is voluntary and cannot be successful unless people start coming to these facilities. Contact tracing which need the sharing of information, access to gated housing societies, reducing the stigmatization of COVID-19 cases and discrimination

---

[16] A. Ghaffar, et al., 'Three way partnerships fuel primary healthcare success', *BMJ Global Health*, 2019: 4.

against healthcare providers is possible only with community participation.

There are many experiences and examples of community participation. At the peak of the pandemic, in urban areas, the Resident Welfare Associations (RWAs) had set up quarantine rooms in the community centres of their societies. In many villages, it was panchayat members who took the initiative in enforcing hygiene and social distancing. During the pandemic, especially in containment zones, the RWAs collaborated with the police to ensure provision of essential services. They facilitated the access of health workers in contact tracing. Many community associations prepared a list of vulnerable and affected individuals. In the beginning of the pandemic, there was a lot of fear and apprehension. It was the power of positive messages from various community representatives and members which helped in reducing the apprehension and allay the fear.

If Kerala succeeded in battling COVID-19 in the early stages of the pandemic, it was because the village panchayat and elected representatives actively participated in the state's response. People helped in contact tracing and slowing down the spread of the virus. In Dharavi, too, as we discussed before, it can largely be attributed to community participation. The slum residents, who were initially reported to be hostile, started coming to fever clinics and volunteering at the quarantine facilities once they trusted the workers. It was a two-way process. It became possible by improving awareness about healthy behaviour as well as delivering essential services to the people in the community. The government gave people what they needed and in return people cooperated.

By mid-July 2020, the Union government released guidelines and standard procedures for effective pandemic response and engagement with the RWAs. There have been many discussions around the world on various facets of community engagement in healthcare services. It has been argued that models could be on a continuum of 'community as recipient of services' to 'community as partner for services'. However, the best approach for community participation would be to have the community be the owner of the response.

Response to the Pandemic during the Unlock

The response to the pandemic has been one of human perseverance and determination. While there have been many cases, many more have been prevented. The country has low case and infection fatality rates (Box 5.4 explains possibly why), which indicates that the response may not have been perfect but it was effective. There have been changes in healthcare systems and services in the four months of unlock from June to September 2020 (see Box 5.5). There are a few learnings that we can take away from the pandemic.

Box 5.4 Why Did India Have Low Case Fatality Rate for COVID-19?

Everyone looked for a scientific explanation for possible low COVID-19 mortality in India. Until May 2020, in many countries, the case fatality rate (CFR), or number of deaths for every 100 confirmed cases, was around 5 to 8 per cent. It was around 3 per cent in India, which further declined.

There were three reasons which were identified as the causes of mortality. First, the agent factor or the virulence or the ability of the virus to cause severe diseases is likely to be similar for all settings and cannot be altered. Second, host factors such as old age and comorbidities or underlying disease conditions such as diabetes, hypertension and other chronic illnesses in any age group were associated with a higher risk. Third, external factors such as insufficient health services and a weak healthcare system can result in increased mortality challenges.

Fortunately, despite several challenges and a population with a high burden of co-morbidities, the mortality figures for India remained relatively low. Public health experts and epidemiologists looked at various possible explanations, including the fact that the average age of the population is young, while mortality is higher in older age groups. Second, there has been some emerging evidence that universal BCG vaccination (for TB) helps in reducing mortality. Third, it was also hypothesized that recurrent infections in a population help in developing an active immune system, which works as a protective shield. It is expected that more learning will evolve on this topic in future.

Box 5.5: Specific Health Initiatives for Pandemic Response, June–September 2020

- The National Clinical Grand Rounds (CGR) on COVID-19 were started by AIIMS, New Delhi, in collaboration with NITI Aayog and MoHFW.
- The number of COVID-19-specific beds were increased to nearly 17 lakh across India for different types of COVID-19 patients.
- The number of COVID-19 testing labs reached 1900 including 45 per cent in the private sector. Around 11 lakh COVID-19 tests are done every day in India.[17]
- India's first I-Lab (infection disease diagnostic lab) for COVID-19 testing in rural and inaccessible areas was launched in June 2020. It has a capacity to test 250 samples through RT-PCR and ELISA.[18]
- A few high throughput laboratories with capacities for nearly 10,000 tests every day have been launched.
- A behaviour change campaign has been launched by NITI Aayog. The information, education and communication (IEC) material was developed and launched for essential focus on mask wearing and hand sanitization.

---

[17] Available at https://www.icmr.gov.in/. Accessed on 2 October 2020.

[18] ELISA: Enzyme-Linked Immunosorbent Assay.

- The National Digital Health Mission (NDHM) was announced by the prime minister on 15 August 2020.
- The National Pharmaceutical Pricing Authority (NPPA) capped the price of medical oxygen when the shortage of oxygen supply was reported.

As with the lockdown, the 'unlock' lasted for four phases, till 30 September 2020. Starting 1 October 2020, the 'reopening' followed 'the unlocks' in India. Around the first week of October 2020, the Nomura India Business Resumption Index was at 82.1, where 100 reflects pre-pandemic level business activity.[19] Clearly, businesses were approaching their normal, but life was yet to return to normal.

[19] Available at https://economictimes.indiatimes.com/news/economy/indicators/business-resumptions-sustained-in-early-october-but-resurging-virus-a-risk-to-growth-nomura/articleshow/78492488.cms.

What Did Everyone Learn during This Period?

- **Implement the known health interventions before searching for new ones.** The experience from the COVID-19 pandemic response in Delhi during June 2020 indicates those interventions which can make a difference.

- **Community participation is integral to health service delivery.** Community engagement is 'an absolute essential' for well-functioning health systems.

- **Strengthening the health system is more than adding beds in the hospitals.** Healthcare is about medical care (curative and diagnostic services) as well as public health services (such as prevention of disease and promotion of health). We need to work on developing a long-lasting and sustainable approach to healthcare.

- **Sustained policy attention and interventions are needed to improve health services.** Elected leaders, health policymakers and subject experts have to regularly intervene and adopt the appropriate local strategies to tackle the same old challenge.

- **Focus on strengthening primary healthcare and public health services.** The COVID-19 pandemic response was more effective in countries with stronger and well-functioning primary healthcare and public health services (e.g. Vietnam and Thailand).

- **There is a need to increase the availability and accessibility to mental health services.** There is a need to rapidly scale up mental health services, preferably through the primary healthcare–based approach. The stigma and discrimination towards patients and healthcare workers are other challenges, waiting for attention.

- **Health and economy are interlinked.** India witnessed a major contraction of the economy in the second quarter of the financial year 2020–21. Much of this was due to slowed-down economic activities due to the pandemic. The interlinkage of health and economy was always known and the pandemic highlighted it once more. It is wise to invest in health to keep the economy growing. The government investment in health is essential for maintaining public health services.

- **Every intervention is part of the solution.** In a pandemic, no single intervention is a complete solution. All of them together work towards defeating the disease.

- **The pandemic will not be over till it is over in all parts of the world.** The duration of the pandemic will depend on combined interventions by policymakers, technical (health and public health) experts and the community at large. It will also depend on how all countries work in solidarity.

6

The Undaunted Human Spirit: Stories from the Frontline

The pandemic has two salutary lessons for societies.

First, it has reminded us who truly keeps society functioning: key workers. Health workers and care workers, shop workers and social workers, bus drivers, teachers, bank tellers, police officers, farmers, and cleaners. Society often takes these workers for granted, but without them, we would sink into chaos.

The second is that society and its systems are much more fragile than many of us appreciated.

The Lancet[1]

In the end, when the history of the COVID-19 pandemic is written, credit would be given to many for battling the

---

[1] 'No more normal', *The Lancet*, Vol. 396, No. 10245: 143. Also available at https://doi.org/10.1016/S0140-6736(20)31591-9.

virus but the maximum space would perhaps be devoted to the frontline workers: doctors, nurses, hospital staff, public health workers, community health workers (majority of whom are women), sanitation workers and everyone who worked directly with those who were infected or could have been infected in the line of duty. In one of its official responses, the government acknowledged that in the fight against COVID-19 in India, by the end of August 2020, nearly 87,000 frontline workers had been affected and nearly 600 of them had died.[2] The actual number could be slightly higher.

In a passionate editorial in the *Hindustan Times*,[3] journalist Karan Thapar wrote: 'As an Army officer's son, I want to frankly say I despair of a society that values its soldiers more than its doctors and nurses. Perhaps that's because of our insecurity. In that case, it could be understandable.' He stressed on the role of the doctors and health workers in fighting a pandemic and the risk they face. He quoted Dr Saleem Naik, who said that 'when a soldier fights a war, it's his own life that's at risk. When doctors, nurses and healthcare staff assist COVID-19 patients, they risk bringing the infection home to their parents, wives and children . . . The enemy's bullet doesn't enter the soldier's household. On

---

[2] Available at https://thefederal.com/covid-19/covid-19-health-workers-pay-price-with-life-for-inadequate-safety-measures/.

[3] Karan Thapar, 'Health Workers: The Soldiers of Our Times'. *The Hindustan Times*, 12 September 2020. Available at https://www.hindustantimes.com/columns/health-workers-the-soldiers-of-our-times-writes-karan-thapar/story-l9R8ehypbyNgm1G0mLYsTP.html.

the other hand, the threat of infection from COVID-19 isn't restricted to hospitals.'

An Unprecedented Challenge and the Response

The assessment of a fight against an enemy has to be context-dependent. COVID-19 has been a pandemic of unprecedented magnitude. No effective vaccine or treatment has yet been found. People without any symptoms are spreading the disease unknowingly. All these factors make its prevention and recovery a challenging task. Even the best of healthcare systems have struggled to contain the virus.

The need for improving India's healthcare system was being discussed even before the pandemic. Yet, when the pandemic happened, there was no choice but to fight. And the Indian healthcare system, despite all the challenges, mounted a concerted response.

The pandemic is being fought by everyone in society. Some were and are in the frontline: the health staff (doctors, nurses, community health workers) as well as essential services workers (police, water supply and electricity supply, and sanitation). It became possible because each one of them was available when and where they were needed and played their roles every single time. The pandemic has underscored the importance of teamwork in healthcare. While public health experts were engaged in planning the response strategy, epidemiologists and researchers attempted to understand the disease pattern. Those in research laboratories started the search for possible therapies and vaccines. Doctors and nurses were involved in medical care and some in the community helped in tracing every contact and following up on anyone who showed symptoms.

Three Government Buildings Where a Lot Was Happening

Many people while crossing the Maulana Azad Road near India Gate in New Delhi do not know that the indistinct Nirman Bhawan building houses the Union ministry of health and family welfare (MoHFW) of the Government of India. It is as easily missed as the National Centre for Disease Control (NCDC) at Shamnath Marg in north Delhi and the Indian Council of Medical Research (ICMR), behind the iconic AIIMS. However, all three of these institutions were the nerve centres of the fight against COVID-19, each looking at some aspects of the country's response. Their focus was on epidemiology, public health and medical care. During the pandemic, these institutions have been as busy on Saturdays and Sundays as if it were a weekday. These offices were not closed even when the entire country was under lockdown. They were clearly the 'essential of the essential services'.

Responding to the COVID-19 pandemic required the engagement of all stakeholders, and every relevant department and institution was involved. The prime minister's office, the ministry of home affairs and NITI Aayog were coordinating many of the responses. However, health was a crucial aspect and the MoHFW was the nodal ministry responsible for it.

At the state level, the departments of health had rarely received the kind of attention as they did during the pandemic. While all sectors worked together, at the state level, the pandemic response was supervised by the offices of the chief ministers as well as the highest levels of administration.

Exposed to Risk Yet Undeterred

Fighting COVID-19 has not been an easy task. Doctors and health staff were working for long hours and at times with very limited resources. Yet, often, even in their normal course of duty, they were abused and harassed. When community-level health workers went to the field for contact tracing, wearing the full PPE in the extreme heat, they were attacked; this happened in different parts of the country, be it Indore in Madhya Pradesh,[4] Munger in Bihar[5] or Bengaluru in Karnataka.[6] Despite this, each one of them continued to do their duty.

There have been many heroes in this fight and many more will emerge in the days to follow. This chapter focuses on a few of them.

---

[4]   Available at https://www.timesnownews.com/india/article/stones-pelted-on-doctors-in-indore-while-tracking-man-who-came-in-contact-with-covid-19-patient-watch/572691.

[5]   Available at https://www.newindianexpress.com/nation/2020/apr/03/health-workers-under-attack-2125058.html.

[6]   Available at https://www.thehindu.com/news/cities/bangalore/they-go-where-others-fear-to-tread/article31428115.ece.

Frontline Workers Who Never Gave Up

Fifty-six-year-old Dr Asheem Gupta was an anaesthesia specialist working in Delhi's Lok Nayak Hospital.[7] A passionate and dedicated doctor, he was involved in fighting COVID-19 from the very beginning. When on 3 May 2020, the Indian Air Force showered flowers over select COVID hospitals across India, a very pleased Dr Gupta told a news channel that though work conditions were difficult, it was the passion to save lives which kept him and his fellow health staff motivated. He succumbed to COVID-19 at the end of June 2020.

Dr U.C. Ghosh was posted at a community clinic in Delhi.[8] He was sixty-five years old. Being at high risk, he was advised by the authorities to go on leave if he wished to do so. However, he chose to continue to work. He got infected and did not survive.

Ambika P.K., a forty-six-year-old nursing officer at a private hospital in Delhi, contracted and died of COVID-19 in the last week of May 2020.[9] Many members of the nursing staff contracted COVID-19 and recovered.

In the second week of July 2020, Constable Yogender Yadav became the twelfth Delhi Police personnel to die of

---

[7] Available at https://theprint.in/india/senior-doctor-at-lnjp-delhis-covid-hospital-dies-days-after-contracting-the-virus/450365/.

[8] Available at https://www.hindustantimes.com/cities/mohalla-clinic-doctor-dies-of-covid-19/story-XvfThrytBpHEIWGJEPZuqK.html.

[9] Available at https://indianexpress.com/article/cities/delhi/46-yr-old-nursing-officer-dies-of-covid-at-safdarjung-6425637/.

COVID-19.[10] Police personnel across the country, be it in Delhi, Mumbai, or any of the other cities, were exposed to and affected by COVID-19. Yet all of them returned to work as soon they recovered.

By the third week of July, it was reported that from health workers to sweepers, nearly 102 Brihanmumbai Municipal Corporation (BMC) workers had died of COVID-19.[11] These included twenty-seven workers from the Solid Waste Management department who collected garbage, including biomedical waste, from assigned areas. Among those who had died were police personnel, community health workers, drivers of essential service vehicles, security guards and sweepers in the hospitals.

Debdutta Roy, the thirty-eight-year-old deputy magistrate of Chandannagar in the Hooghly district of West Bengal, was in charge of Shramik Express trains, which were ferrying the returning migrants to their homes.[12] She was also in charge of managing everything at the quarantine centres for the migrant labourers who had returned. In the course of her work, she was exposed to the virus and tested positive. She did not survive.

---

[10] Available at https://indianexpress.com/article/cities/delhi/cop-dies-of-covid-leaves-2-kids-behind-6496996/.

[11] Available at https://indianexpress.com/article/cities/mumbai/health-worker-to-sweeper-some-of-102-bmc-workers-who-died-of-covid-6517230/.

[12] Available at https://indianexpress.com/article/cities/kolkata/bengal-covid-19-caseload-up-to-31448-senior-district-official-among-24-dead-6504561/.

These are stories that are representative of the many doctors, nurses, health workers and other essential services workers, who risked and continue to risk their lives to save people.

When Protecting and Saving Lives Is the Only Purpose

Dr Zahid Abdul Majeed, wearing the PPE coveralls, was with a patient who was being transferred to the ICU. Suddenly he noticed that the intubation (a procedure where a tube is placed in the trachea in the neck of a person to ensure breathing) pipe had been displaced. This could have been life-threatening for the patient. The PPE along with the face cover blurred his vision, which was not good enough to conduct a complex procedure to reposition the intubation pipe. Dr Majeed took off his protective gear and re-intubated the patient.[13] This was in the line of his duty, where he risked his own life to save the life of a patient. He was sent for a mandatory isolation of fourteen days, as per standard procedure. His story is the story of hundreds of health workers fighting every single day in India, and across the world.

A nursing staff from a leading nursing home said, 'I, along with others, received an hour-long training and was soon posted to the [COVID-19] ward. Initially, there was clarity on very few things. Nearly all of us had fears, everyone,

---

[13] Available at https://www.thehindu.com/news/cities/Delhi/aiims-doctor-removes-safety-gear-risks-life-to-save-covid-19-patient/article31552814.ece.

doctors, nurses and other staff. Initially, there were just a few patients, but soon the number of patients increased and the load per doctor and nursing staff went up as well. There were many serious patients. It causes a lot of mental stress. Our family members remain worried. But they know this is war. And soldiers do not run away in a war. They fight till the end. I will also do the same.'[14]

Women Power: Frontline Fighters in Communities

India's fight against COVID-19 at the frontline has been led by nearly 3.6 million women workers, which includes 900,000 ASHA workers, 200,000 auxiliary nurse midwives (ANMs), 1.3 million AWWs and 1.2 million Anganwadi helpers, and many others. During these months of the pandemic, they touched several lives, directly and indirectly.

Most of these workers received some handouts and underwent short training sessions at the beginning of the pandemic. Ever since then, they have been working every single day to help the country respond to the pandemic. ASHA workers have visited, on an average, twenty-five houses every day, prepared the list of people in the houses and advised them on what to do if anyone was at high risk or had symptoms. In a news story in *The Hindu*,[15] one ASHA worker described herself as a drone to the Kerala Police. In

---

[14] As told to the authors.
[15] Available at https://www.thehindu.com/society/at-the-forefront-of-indias-healthcare-system-asha-workers-soldier-on-unprotected-and-poorly-paid/article31979010.ece.

disease surveillance for influenza-like illnesses (ILI) and SARI, they were the ones providing exact and accurate information to the authorities to act on. Contact tracing, house-to-house surveys and other field activities which were being conducted in order to respond effectively to the pandemic would have been impossible if it were not for the ASHAs and AWWs.

These women workers have faced many struggles in their work. Like all other health workers at the frontline, there have been reports of deaths and COVID-19 infection among ASHA workers. These workers do not get a fixed monthly salary and there have also been reports of delay in their payments. The courts have intervened and argued for them and on behalf of all health workers, saying 'in a war, one cannot have unhappy soldiers'.[16] There have been frequent reports of these workers being boycotted by the village for being a potential source of infection. There have been many reported instances where their neighbours started avoiding meeting or interacting with them.

The response to the pandemic is largely dependent on awareness, behaviour modification and the education of the public. People need up-to-date and correct information (and not the kind which is circulated on social media platforms). Throughout the pandemic one heard of the heroic efforts of frontline healthcare workers contributing on various fronts of the pandemic. There were many stories in the media. These included the stories of an ASHA worker in Assam who overcame enormous challenges, including floods, and

---

[16] Available at https://timesofindia.indiatimes.com/india/in-war-you-dont-make-soldiers-unhappy-sc-on-non-payment-of-salaries-to-doctors/articleshow/76336942.cms.

ensured that people received the health services they needed. As the country continues with a long struggle to respond to the pandemic, the role of the frontline warrior becomes more and more important. This is clearly a case for treating frontline workers with the dignity and respect they deserve.[17]

Contributions of People from Every Walk of Life

Various agencies, institutes and organizations reprioritized their roles and resources to ensure they contributed to the pandemic response. In the course of the pandemic, a few Indian newspapers[18] have[19] documented the stories of kindness and positivity, which emerged from nearly every part of the country.

In March 2020, the National Institute of Mental Health and Neuro-Sciences (NIMHANS), Bengaluru, set up a 24x7 call centre to provide counselling to people in distress. Since then, several thousand calls have been responded to during the pandemic by trained psychiatrists, psychologists and other counsellors.[20] NIMHANS has connected with nearly

---

[17] Available at https://www.hindustantimes.com/analysis/why-society-owes-asha-workers-a-debt/story-sKhgxsrNcH9mShfVhYaFzL.html.

[18] Available at https://indianexpress.com/facebook-stories-of-strength-2020/.

[19] Available at https://www.hindustantimes.com/topic/ht-salute.

[20] Available at https://indianexpress.com/article/facebook-stories-of-strength-2020/case-studies/trying-to-calm-nerves-24x7-this-team-at-nimhans-needs-nerves-of-steel-6431574/.

130 mental healthcare professionals to help people in need of mental health services.

Doctors for You, a small non-governmental organization ensured that volunteers as well as doctors and nurses were available wherever needed. They engaged with governments for setting up isolation and quarantine centres in a few cities and states of India. Community-based organizations such as the Lok Swasthya Sewa Trust and Ekjut continued to work, during the lockdown and afterwards, with women at the grassroots level and the rural population to generate awareness about diseases, address mental health issues and to facilitate access to health services. They used the presence of volunteers at the grassroots level and also delivered messages over phone calls. The period also witnessed innovative mobile-based applications which were used by families and people at large. These are some examples of the small contributions made by select organizations; but similar contributions by thousands of such organizations helped make a difference.

In May 2020, a gurudwara in Nanded, Maharashtra, made headlines for the wrong reasons. Many pilgrims who had been stranded there during the lockdown and had returned to their homes in Punjab tested positive for COVID-19. However, in the weeks to follow, the gurudwara committee handed over the same building, where the pilgrims had been housed, to the district administration, to convert it to a CCC. Soon, it started housing COVID-19 patients.[21] Food for all

---

[21] Available at https://indianexpress.com/article/india/maharashtra-nanded-gurdwaras-now-covid-care-centres-6437965/.

patients at this facility was provided free of cost through the langar in the gurudwara.

Radha Soami Satsang Beas in Chhatarpur, Delhi, offered to prepare and distribute free meals to all the patients admitted to the 10,000-bed COVID-19-care facility which was set up to tackle the peak in Delhi in June 2020.

There are innumerable such positive stories. A group of women in Arunachal Pradesh served hot meals to frontline workers to ensure that none of them went hungry at work. The patients who had tested negative and recovered returned to COVID-19 facilities to donate convalescent plasma and save lives. The mortuary staff in hospitals overstayed a few hours every day to dispose of the additional dead bodies. Junior doctors who were on leave to prepare for their final exams, which would have determined whether they would get their degree or not, returned to work, as saving lives was more important. Health staff overstayed beyond their working hours to ensure that every patient got the best possible service, irrespective of the challenges. Many young engineers and graduate students contributed to develop mobile applications to track the disease and address the 'infodemic' (the information epidemic made it a challenging task to separate reliable information from rumours).[22] An employee of a leading publishing house initiated crowdfunding to send grocery items for all those in need.

---

[22] Available at https://www.who.int/news/item/23-09-2020-managing-the-covid-19-infodemic-promoting-healthy-behaviours-and-mitigating-the-harm-from-misinformation-and-disinformation.

Several ASHA workers in different parts of the country left their young children at home and headed out in the field to respond to the pandemic. They conducted house-to-house surveys in containment zones, traced contacts, and identified those with early-stage symptoms. An Anganwadi worker in Bihar suffered from a leg injury. That did not deter her from doing her duty. She regularly conducted door-to-door COVID-19 health surveys in her area.[23]

A fifty-six-year-old employee of a state government was the in-charge and warden of a temporary shelter home in a school.[24] In April 2020, during the lockdown, this shelter home housed over 400 people. Every day, this employee worked at the shelter home from 8 a.m. to 10 p.m. and refused to take leave. In Mumbai, a thirty-five-year-old auto driver set up a community kitchen which prepared meals for 250 to 300 people every day. The meals were for migrant workers and labourers stranded due to the lockdown.[25]

There are stories of families of doctors, where each member was involved in fighting COVID-19. There are stories of patients who donated convalescent plasma more

---

[23] Available at https://www.hindustantimes.com/india-news/leg-injury-doesn-t-stop-govt-worker-from-carrying-out-health-surveys/story-zR89KV5CEexfUAMgwDnznK.html.

[24] Available at https://www.hindustantimes.com/india-news/ht-salutes-refused-to-take-leave-works-14-hour-days/story-UbJrTCGROseO0y4UofomSM.html.

[25] Available at https://www.hindustantimes.com/india-news/mumbai-s-autodriver-sets-up-community-kitchen-in-covid-affected-area/story-6j5hsjeu68JQFi8oAeN3NI.html

than once to ensure that all those who needed the potentially life-saving investigational therapy had access to it.

The pandemic needed everyone to play their respective role. However, societal biases did not spare anyone. In June 2020, a security guard posted at one of Delhi's leading government hospitals was attacked with bricks by neighbours who accused him of spreading the virus. This was not an isolated incident and many similar reports came to light from different parts of the country.

When additional resources were needed for an intensified COVID-19 response, many more people joined the effort. The door-to-door surveys brought together booth-level officers, volunteers, teachers and police constables. In fact, schoolteachers played multiple roles in the fight against COVID-19. They were part of community surveys in a few places that facilitated activities related to the setting up of quarantine centres.

During the pandemic, schools played a new role. Initially, many schools served as a place to shelter migrants. Schools were among the places where food was prepared and distributed. Later on, state-government-run schools became quarantine facilities and, subsequently, many schools were converted to CCCs.

Panchayat members and representatives across many parts of India initiated proactive action to generate awareness about the coronavirus to promote healthy behaviour among people; they also made necessary arrangements for returning migrants. States such as Odisha empowered the panchayats with several rights, including the authority to enforce a lockdown in their zone. It was widely reported that wherever the panchayat played an active role, the spread of the disease was slower.

India, a Country of and Built by Internal Migrants

In April and May 2020, the visuals of migrants returning to their homes on foot were among the most defining images of the pandemic in India. The plight of migrant workers highlighted the social impact of disease and pandemics on human life. As migrants attempted to reach their home cities, they were kept at various quarantined centres set up in community halls, empty training centres, and schools. In a city in Rajasthan, migrants were quarantined in a school. While in quarantine, the migrants helped paint the school building. When they left, the school building was in a far better condition than before.

The story of migrants is also that of resilience. When the 'unlock' started and business activities resumed, migrants were back in demand. The ones who happened to stay back in Delhi helped in setting up a 10,000-bed CCC in a short period of time. In fact, nearly 900 workers, mostly migrants, worked in multiple shifts to ensure the timely completion of this facility.

All Heroes Do Not Wear Capes

We have seen the images of COVID-19 patients, in a happy mood, sitting comfortably in COVID-19 facilities playing a game of chess. We have read stories of doctors, nurses, police personnel and other frontline workers returning to their duties soon after recovering from their illness. Personal tragedies, challenges and struggles notwithstanding, all of us can do something for another. This is how the pandemic has been fought so far by everyone in India. There are heroes all around us, thousands and millions, who just don't happen to wear capes. These are people from all walks of life who are working to defeat the virus and stop the pandemic. All we have to do is recognize these 'heroes without capes' and give them their due respect and recognition, every single time, always.

What Did Everyone Learn during This Period?

- **Health workers are vital for the functioning of health services.** Health is part of the service sector, which is dependent on human resources. In all parts of the world, a large proportion of the total expenditure on health is on the salaries of the staff. When there is underinvestment in health services, there is a shortage of qualified and trained staff. It affects the motivation of the staff members and adversely affects their retention in the health system and thus the availability of health services. India needs to increase government funding for health and make policies to ensure equitable distribution and retention of health staff.

- **Community health workers are the foundation of health systems.** There are a few million community health workers in India, who act as a bridge between community members and healthcare facilities. They are the face of health services to the people. They deliver information and offer many preventive and promotive healthcare services. They have a role in converting a 'medical care' system into a 'healthcare' system.

- **Engage, recruit and post a wide range of healthcare staff beyond doctors and nurses.** The delivery of health services needs a broader range of health staff. It should involve epidemiologists, public health specialists, laboratory technicians, pharmacists, counsellors, community health workers and many other allied health staff. Each one of them is needed to ensure delivery of the entire range of preventive, promotive, curative, diagnostic, and rehabilitative and palliative care services.

- **Take initiatives for infection prevention and control.** The safety of health workers and provision for infection prevention and control at the health facilities will make the healthcare services safe and effective from the perspective of both the health staff and the patients.

- **It needs teamwork to keep society healthy.** COVID-19 has taught us once again that health is more than medical care. Other sectors have a role to play as well. For instance, within the healthcare sector there are multiple agencies delivering health services, such as local corporations, and Union and state government agencies. There is also a need for inter-sectoral collaboration (with institutions associated with nutrition, water supply and sanitation, and so on; in other words, those looking after the social determinants of health. Mechanisms for teamwork and collaborative engagements need to be strengthened and institutionalized.

Section III

Science, Solidarity and Hope

The period following the declaration of COVID-19 as a pandemic has been an interesting and perhaps even an exciting time for the general public who are getting to see how science advances and works. The early findings of scientific research are being published in newspapers and discussed by everyone, from news anchors to students. What is a clinical trial? Why do doctors not know what to use? If a drug works in one trial, why does it not work in another? How are results shared? Why do treatment protocols vary in different countries?

The names of reputed international medical journals such as *The Lancet* and *The New England Journal of Medicine* have by now been heard by many non-medical persons for the first time. The constant barrage of information at times also created confusion for many people. A treatment which seemed to have worked based on initial studies failed in subsequent well-conducted trials. People are closely watching every development on vaccines and the various steps in vaccine research. They now have a better understanding of how trials are conducted and the fallacies of over-interpreting the results of small not-so-well-conducted studies. Journalists and the public in general discuss articles based on pre-release data even before they are peer reviewed or published. Often this results in a premature hope that a treatment has finally been found. However, more and more of us have by now realized the complexities of clinical trials and the challenges in interpreting the data. Research, globally, has now come to centre stage.

Science has been the real reason for hope during the pandemic.

7

Drugs and Therapies: In Search of Effective Treatment

Can the world win the fight against the pandemic without proven therapies and safe and effective vaccines? Will the pandemic be over when vaccines are available? How are herd immunity and vaccination linked? These were, among many others, questions that experts had deliberated over the years in their attempt to warn the world about epidemics or pandemics. Particularly regarding pandemics, while it was agreed that they were very likely to happen, it was thought that the next big pandemic would be that of influenza. Having handled SARS, MERS and H1N1 in the past twenty years, perhaps we had reassured ourselves that we had the knowledge and technology to quickly control any pandemic. However, when COVID-19 emerged, we had no therapy and no vaccine. The initial response to the COVID-19 pandemic, in all parts of the world, was based on scientific understanding and prior experience of infectious diseases and viruses, and public health. A few months into the pandemic, empirical response (those based on past experience and expert opinion) is slowly being replaced by evidence-based approaches as we learn more about the disease. Science and evidence-based research is now taking shape in all aspects of pandemic response.

What Happens When There Is No Known Treatment Available?

Recall the last time you had fever and cough and visited a doctor. It was probably a ten- or fifteen-minute interaction, during which the doctor would have advised you to take rest and drink plenty of water. The doctor may also have prescribed a few pills (not necessarily an antibiotic) to reduce the symptoms.

It is also possible that if you had an illness which may have been spread by coughing and sneezing, the doctor would have advised you to cover your mouth while coughing. No matter which part of the country (or world) you are in, it is likely that you would be provided a similar course of treatment, with minor variations. A standardized approach is how medical science functions and it is backed by current evidence on how best to manage such a clinical situation.

In the early couple of months of 2020, when the COVID-19 pandemic was spreading across the world, there was limited consensus on the range of symptoms. We knew little else than that the infection was respiratory and could be severe. Laboratory tests were quickly developed but there was limited availability of the testing services. There was no proven effective treatment.

'Empirical Treatment' as the Best Strategy

What therapeutic approach is followed when a new disease appears and there is no known treatment? The first thought is to treat the symptoms; second, to follow an empirical approach, in other words, what is considered logical and appropriate, applying scientific principles. Most COVID-19 patients suffered from fever and cough, and the symptoms were mild. From a clinical perspective, they were put under close medical watch, given medicines to reduce fever, and treated for any change in clinical condition. From a public health perspective, the experiences being reported from Wuhan had already revealed the need for isolation.

A small proportion of COVID-19 cases had difficulty in breathing (or breathlessness). In such cases, usually due to pneumonia or micro-clots in the vessels of the lungs, the oxygen saturation in the blood of the person would start to decline, at times quite suddenly. In these cases, the oxygen saturation needed to be closely monitored. It should be 95 per cent or higher. If the oxygen saturation fell below 95 per cent, it was a sign that close observation and supplemental oxygen might be required. Such patients were classified as moderate cases. At least initially in China, patients with breathing difficulty were put on ventilators quickly, but within a couple of months doctors realized that early invasive ventilation was not required. For those with SARS-CoV-2 infection, it was discovered that simple oxygen could indeed be life-saving. It was thus crucially important for healthcare centres treating COVID-19 to have an adequate supply of oxygen. Since the oxygen saturation of affected individuals needed to be regularly monitored, the need for the wider use of pulse oximeters was identified. If the saturation did not improve with oxygen given through a mask or with a cannula or a plastic tube, high-flow nasal oxygen (HFNO) therapy or a non-invasive ventilation (NIV) approach was used at healthcare facilities. Only two to three out of every ten patients who developed symptoms would reach this stage.

Apart from these observations, it was recognized that making patients lie in the prone position—on their bellies—could improve their oxygen saturation levels. This method, termed 'proning', had been used in the past in the ICU for patients on mechanical ventilators who were not maintaining adequate saturation; it had been found to be effective in clinical trials. However, before COVID-19, 'proning' was not done with conscious patients. This process came to be known as 'conscious proning' and many patients whose oxygen was low were asked to lie on their side and on their belly. This allows the base of the lungs, especially the lung on the posterior side to expand more freely and take in more oxygen and thereby improve oxygen saturation. This benefitted many individuals and helped avoid the need for ventilators either partly or entirely. Though more studies are needed to ascertain exactly how many this approach has benefitted, and how it works, it is considered potentially useful and is now routinely used in most hospitals.

While these measures work in a large proportion of the cases, there are a few whose health condition continues to deteriorate. Such cases are classified as severe and need to be admitted to specialized health facilities or hospitals where there is provision for ICUs and ventilators. Not all these patients necessarily need ICUs and ventilators, but keeping them in such equipped facilities when admitted reduces the delay in transferring them to places with these facilities in case their condition worsens.

Those admitted in the ICU are observed and monitored closely. Their vital parameters such as blood pressure, heart rate, breathing rate and urine output are monitored. A proportion of those in the ICU need to be put on assisted or mechanical ventilation. In such cases, the person's lungs are not functioning well: they are either not able to help in gas exchange (take in oxygen into the blood and expel carbon dioxide) or not able to suck air into the lungs due to fatigue in the breathing muscles (respiratory failure).

The machines which help the breathing process in such a scenario are called ventilators. When an individual is on a ventilator, the machine essentially breathes for him/her, pushing in oxygen and removing carbon dioxide at a set rate and volume. Ventilators are complex devices as they have to push oxygen carefully into the unhealthy and fragile lung, making sure that they do not cause more damage, a complication called ventilator-induced lung injury (VILI). These devices need constant adjustment as the patient's needs change depending on how the disease evolves with time. This device is an essential tool for severe respiratory illnesses. Patients in severe respiratory distress may need to have a ventilator breathe for them until their lungs heal.

However, the ICU is just a well-equipped hospital set-up for intensive monitoring and management. Ventilators are machines which support treatment until the patient recovers the ability to breathe. Therefore, essentially, treatment for COVID-19 has been centred on providing good supportive care. None of these is specific treatment for the disease itself.

To facilitate recovery from diseases, the virus needs to be cleared from the body of the affected person. Moreover, the effects caused by the viral infection, such as an increased clotting mechanism or a hyper-inflammatory response, need to be reversed. Recovery or return to health, therefore, involves reversal of all clinical conditions triggered by the virus.

In any infectious disease, in order to prevent it from progressing to the severe stage, first the cause of the infection needs to be addressed and then the body's response to the infection. The primary focus is on stopping the multiplication of the virus. However, since the SARS-CoV-2 virus was not known earlier, how could any specific drug have been developed? When the pandemic emerged, we did not have a medicine available.

Give Me Any Therapy, Urgently!

In the early period of the pandemic, especially in March–April 2020, in a few countries, nearly one in every ten to twenty patients (or 5 to 10 per cent of total identified cases) had died.[1] This was a high mortality rate. A treatment was urgently needed.

---

[1] Available at https://www.worldometers.info/coronavirus/coronavirus-death-rate/.

There are standard procedures for research on drugs and therapies and for making these available for use. There is a process that is to be followed before a doctor can prescribe a medicine.

First, a potential biochemical or biologic molecule is identified. The initial in-vitro ('in glass', meaning, in a laboratory) studies are done, which are followed by preclinical trials on animals, which can look either for toxic side effects or for treatment in a model of the disease. Once the molecule is found to be non-toxic and effective on animal models, clinical trials on humans are started. Once all phases of the clinical trials are conducted as per the protocol agreed on, and if the drug is found to be safe and effective, it is submitted to the regulatory authorities for a review. After a thorough review, if it meets the criteria of quality, safety and efficacy for licensing, the drug is approved. It is after this process of testing and approval that production is started and a drug becomes available for prescription and sale. Needless to say, drug research takes years, with no one being certain about the final outcome. (Nearly similar steps are followed for vaccine research and development). Many molecules which show potential in preclinical trials fail in clinical trials due to lack of significant efficacy or unacceptable side effects.

SARS-CoV-2 is a virus and there are not many effective therapies against viruses. There are many existing medications against bacteria, called antibiotics. The first antibiotic was developed in the mid-1940s; however, the first antiviral—acyclovir—was developed in the early 1970s. The HIV/AIDS pandemic resulted in an intensive research for drugs. Yet, it took many years before the first effective anti-HIV drug could be made available. Since then, we have learnt a great deal about the disease, and there are many drugs against HIV. Also, by applying the HIV experience to other viruses, we are getting better at making antivirals. Very recently, effective antivirals have been found against the hepatitis C virus, which are actually curing a disease that killed many just a few years ago. However, there are not as many antivirals as there are antibacterial drugs, and the timelines for development and testing are long. Yet, there have been successes.

During any pandemic, time is a luxury. Clearly, the first option was the repurposing of drugs. Scientist started looking for already existing therapies in early 2020 which had either suggested efficacy with similar respiratory viral infections or had shown some benefit with other coronavirus infections.

Hope Pinned on a Seventy-Five-Year-Old Drug: Hydroxychloroquine

Malaria, known to humans for centuries, affects millions of people every year and kills thousands across the world. However, an effective drug—chloroquine—was discovered only in 1930. This life-saving medicine significantly contributed to reducing deaths caused by malaria. As with all drugs, it had some side effects. However, since malaria was a dreadful disease, the side-effects of chloroquine were considered minor in comparison and it began to be used widely.

Alongside, a search for another medicine with fewer side effects continued. In 1946, hydroxychloroquine (HCQ) was invented as a less toxic version of chloroquine. HCQ also had side effects, but these were rarer and it was better tolerated by patients. Since then, HCQ has been used to treat malaria as well as serving as a preventive therapy or a prophylactic for travellers to malaria-endemic regions.

All drugs act by a certain mechanism, and sometimes one drug can be used for multiple diseases. In the case of HCQ, the anti-inflammatory and immune-suppressant properties began to be used to treat autoimmune disorders such as systemic lupus erythematosus (SLE) and rheumatoid arthritis (RA). In many countries where there is no malaria, HCQ is exclusively used for treating SLE and RA by the rheumatologists (the doctors who specialize in joint-related disorders).

In the beginning of the COVID-19 pandemic, epidemiologists were trying to identify patterns of the disease and a potential treatment. From China there were reports that patients with rheumatoid disorders were relatively less affected. Preliminary analysis noted that COVID-19 infections were relatively less in those who were regularly taking HCQ than those who were not. It was due to this information and analysis that doctors felt that HCQ might have the potential to prevent or cure COVID-19. There were a few early studies from China on the use of HCQ for COVID-19 which also indicated that it was useful.

French scientists had been using HCQ for a bacterial infection called 'Q fever'. There had also been some laboratory evidence on that drug acting effectively against SARS-CoV-2. Soon, French researchers reported early evidence in a small number of patients that HCQ (in combination with other medicines) could reduce the duration of viral load and virus shedding[2] in the upper respiratory tract.[3]

In India, HCQ was included as a prophylactic measure for healthcare workers dealing with patients and for those coming into close contact with COVID-19 patients, and later on, as a prophylactic for all frontline workers dealing with COVID-19 cases. Many countries started using HCQ either as a treatment or for prophylaxis or both. Scientists and clinicians continued to debate the value of empirical approaches.

Recognizing that this approach needed to be backed by evidence, the drug was included in number of clinical trials including the RECOVERY trial in the UK and the Solidarity trial led by the WHO. In approximately five weeks: from the third week of May 2020 to the end of June 2020, the fortune of HCQ fluctuated. By the end of May, two research papers published in two high-end medical journals, *The Lancet* and *The New England Journal of Medicine* (NEJM), published articles arguing against the use of HCQ.[4] Within a few days, experts pointed out several

---

[2] Viral load reflects the amount of virus present in a person's body, when the person is infected. Virus shedding is indicative of how much virus is being released from the mouth and the nose. Both of these are dependent on many factors including an individual's immune response.

[3] Available at https://www.sciencedirect.com/science/article/pii/ S1477893920302179.

[4] M.R. Mehra, et al., (Retracted) 'Hydroxychloroquine or Chloroquine with or without a Macrolide for Treatment of COVID-19: A Multinational Registry Analysis', *The Lancet*,

loopholes in the papers. The papers were retracted from both the journals, which meant the papers were considered unpublished and the findings were not to be considered in future. This was unprecedented.

HCQ was back in the game and continued to be used in trials. There was great hope, but it did not last long. The interim analysis of data from the RECOVERY trial in the UK (more on this later) did not find any benefit of HCQ in comparison to those who were not given HCQ. In mid-October 2020, the data from the WHO-led Solidarity trial in nearly thirty countries found that HCQ was not useful in the treatment of COVID-19 among hospitalized patients. Large studies, therefore, did not support the initial enthusiasm for HCQ as a cheap and effective drug that could work against COVID-19. Other smaller trials using HCQ for prophylaxis also showed that the drug was ineffective. All this highlights why the generation of real evidence, with scientific rigour, is a cornerstone of modern medicine. We start with what we know, and try to use it for the benefit of patients, while testing the drug in a range of conditions. If the results show that the drug works, then it will be widely recommended and become the 'standard of care', and if the drug does not work, it will be discarded.

22 May 2020:S0140-6736(20)31180-6, DOI: 10.1016/S0140-6736(20)31180-6.

M.R. Mehra, et al., (Retracted) 'Cardiovascular Disease, Drug Therapy, and Mortality in COVID-19', *NEJM*, 25 June 2020;382(26):2582. DOI: 10.1056/NEJMc2021225. Epub 4 June 2020.

The Repurposing of Drugs

As finding a new drug immediately for a novel virus that was making people sick was not an option, medical experts had to rely on the second-best option at hand: the use of available drugs. This approach is called 'repurposing of drugs'. It is not as easy it may appear to be. A medicine or therapy can be used only for the purpose for which it has been approved. Its use for a new condition requires fresh approval by the regulatory authorities. In these cases, the necessary approvals are sought with a sound rationale for the proposed repurposing. Even during an outbreak, such approvals are granted only after an expedited review process by the national regulatory authorities, which are responsible for ensuring that only safe and effective drugs are used in a country. When drugs are approved so quickly, they are approved as 'emergency use authorization' or EUA, and are subject to further reviews as additional evidence becomes available.

HCQ was not the only drug in which hope was placed. The other drugs which received a lot of attention were the licensed anti-HIV drug, lopinavir-ritonavir and the antiviral drug remdesivir. Lopinavir-ritonavir was reported to be useful in China and promoted as being effective against COVID-19, but subsequently in well-designed clinical trials, including the WHO Solidarity study, it did not show any benefit. The drug is no longer being used.[5]

---

5   B. Cao, et al., 'A Trial of Lopinavir–Ritonavir in Adults Hospitalized with Severe COVID-19', *NEJM*, 2020.

Remdesivir was first developed in 2014 to treat Ebola and was subsequently also explored as a treatment against the hepatitis C virus and MERS. A research paper published in April 2020 indicated that remdesivir was able to inhibit the virus and prevent further spread.[6] Remdesivir was 'repurposed' in the fight against COVID-19. It was included in a number of drug trials including the Solidarity trial, DisCoVeRy trial, one large trial in the US, and two in China. Early results from a study supported by the US National Institutes of Health had shown that remdesivir could reduce the recovery time of people hospitalized with COVID-19 from fifteen to eleven days.[7]

However, in the Solidarity trial, remdesivir did not show any effect on progression to ventilation or mortality. This can seem complicated because some trials show a positive result and others do not. But a lot depends on when the drugs are used—early in the disease or late—and what results are being measured: whether it is an effect on the virus ('shedding'), on the disease—which is measured by clinical estimations of how the patient is doing—or on the prevention of death.

---

[6] Y. Wang, et al., 'Remdesivir in Adults with Severe COVID-19: A Randomised, Double-Blind, Placebo-Controlled, Multicentre Trial', *The Lancet*, 2020; 1569–78. First published on 29 April 2020. Available at https://www.thelancet.com/journals/lancet/ article/PIIS0140-6736(20)31022-9/fulltext. Accessed on 15 September 2020.

[7] J.H. Beigel, et al., 'Remdesivir for the Treatment of COVID-19— Preliminary Report', *NEJM*, 22 May 2020. DOI: 10.1056/ NEJMoa2007764. Accessed on 15 September 2020.

The drugs controller general of India has approved emergency-use authorization for remdesivir.[8] It is recommended for moderately to severely ill patients.

Besides these drugs, many physicians started 'off-label, use[9] of other drugs based on small studies which suggested some antiviral activity of the drug against COVID-19. This included drugs like ivermectin and favipiravir. Since drugs which are approved have been tested for safety, physicians use their experience to tailor treatments for their patients. This is acceptable in the early stages, but to generate additional evidence that a drug really does work for the purpose for which it is being used, clinical trials are required.

Drug Research and Trials: Global Collaboration and Indian Participation

It was clear that finding a new molecule for effective treatment would be a far slower process than repurposing of drugs and putting them into clinical trials. Let's take the example of 'proning'—globally, clinicians have reported proning to have shown a beneficial effect, but it has not been evaluated in a clinical trial. Randomly allocating patients for prone positioning has ethical and scientific issues in the design

---

[8] Available at https://pib.gov.in/PressReleasePage.aspx?PRID= 1631509.

[9] This refers to the use of a drug for a disease condition for which it was not originally approved or its use in a formulation different than originally approved. Available at https://www.fda.gov/patients/ learn-about-expanded-access-and-other-treatment-options/ understanding-unapproved-use-approved-drugs-label.

and conduct of clinical trials. Yet, the risk to the patients by changing their position to make breathing easier is low and, therefore, it has been widely used. However, drugs are a different ball game. They need to be tested in clinical trials, and should not be used without conducting studies. With drugs, there is a risk of false assurance that a treatment works and is safe, while the truth may be otherwise. 'Do no harm' is the dictum which must always be followed. Proven therapies should be used, while unproven ones must be discarded.

One of the problems with finding new treatments for SARS-CoV-2 was that with a new virus that no one understood, there was a desperation in the medical community to get something that worked to help their patients. In China, within the first six weeks of the pandemic, over 120 clinical trials were planned and begun.

A simple explanation of a clinical trial is that if we want to test a new treatment, it is given to half of the total number of patients in the trial who have the disease, the other half gets a placebo, that is a drug that appears, tastes and smells like the new treatment but in reality does not have it. To make sure that there is no bias in testing the new treatment, the investigational drug and the placebo are administered using a number of ways to ensure that the researcher cannot decide which particular patient gets the treatment and who gets the placebo—these processes are called random allocation and blinding. This ensures that when improvements (or the lack of them) are measured, there will be no bias because no one will know who got the trial treatment and who got the placebo until the trial is over and the results are available for a comparison of the two arms, often termed the 'treatment and control' arms of the trial.

There are many other considerations that are important in clinical trials including the stage of illness, the location, how many drugs are being studied, what kinds of tests are used, what is the outcome based on which it will be decided whether the new treatment worked or not, and, most importantly, in how many people should the study be done so that we can be sure that this new treatment will work in most settings and disease states in the real world. If the trial is done in too few people, it is a waste, because the results will need to be reproduced in many trials before we can be confident that the results are reliable and we can use the drug. Most of the 120 trials conducted in China, led to no useful results because they were too small. Unfortunately, we have seen the same picture in India and elsewhere, with many, many small trials being conducted which are unlikely to lead to any conclusions that will reliably tell us what works and what does not for COVID-19 patients.

Thankfully, there have also been more sensible approaches. Because trials and evidence were needed from different settings and countries, and the pandemic differed in intensity from region to region across the world, at times recruiting enough patients quickly for a trial became a challenge. To address this, the WHO initiated a large multinational trial called the Solidarity trial in many hospitals in many countries in the world. The trial had a simple design with a focus not on gathering the very detailed data usually collected on each patient in a trial, but to get only the key outcomes: did the patient get worse as measured by needing ventilation, did the patient better and get discharged or did the patient die? Additionally, the trial was designed to use the drugs available in each country, so that the results could be used quickly by doctors in that country.

The first drugs studied in the Solidarity trial were HCQ, lopinavir-ritonavir, with and without interferon, and remdesivir. Another large trial was started in the UK. This was made possible by the fact that hospitals in the UK are a part of the National Health Service. Therefore, instead of many small trials, one large trial could be done. This was the RECOVERY (Randomized Evaluation of COVID-19 therapy) Trial[10] and focused on low-dose dexamethasone, azithromycin, tocilizumab and convalescent plasma, in different arms of the trial (which means different patients received one of these therapies). It was the result from this trial which led to the recommendation of dexamethasone as a treatment for COVID-19. The trial of treatments for COVID-19 in hospitalized adults (DisCoVeRy)[11] was led by an institute of the French government, and had interventions similar to the Solidarity trial that focused on remdesivir, lopinavir-ritonavir, interferon beta 1A and HCQ. This trial contributed its data to the analysis of the Solidarity trial.

The observations made during the first few months of the pandemic have underscored the importance of drugs and clinical research and development. By the end of September 2020, many therapies and treatments, including many traditional medicines, were being explored. Of all these,

---

[10] Available at https://www.recoverytrial.net/.

[11] Available at https://clinicaltrials.gov/ct2/show/NCT04315948.

steroids like dexamethasone and methylprednisolone in patients in need of supplemental oxygen or on a ventilator as well as anticoagulants had shown to have a beneficial effect.[12] In mid-October 2020, the findings of the Solidarity trial were released and unfortunately none of the four therapies were found to show any beneficial effect on COVID-19 treatment in severely ill patients.[13] This means that we still do not have a specific antiviral drug against COVID-19 and the key management strategy has to be good supportive care with oxygen and steroids when indicated and as per treatment protocols.

When the Human Immune System Overreacts

It has been proposed that one of the key responses in some patients of COVID-19, especially those with a severe form of the disease, is an excessive release of cytokines. Cytokines are inflammatory markers produced in the body which act as a signal to the human immune system to fight foreign particles and pathogens. Cytokines trigger the immune system to respond to any threat. They are part of the body's immune response to fight off any infection, including COVID-19. When there is excessive release of these markers, it is called a 'cytokine storm'. When this happens, the ability of the body to differentiate between its own cells and foreign cells

---

[12] Available at https://www.nytimes.com/interactive/2020/science/coronavirus-drugs-treatments.html.

[13] Available at https://www.medrxiv.org/content/10.1101/2020.10.15.20209817v1.

nearly disappears. The situation is often compared with an indiscriminate firing in a public place where a lot of collateral damage happens. At this stage, rather than being protective, a person's immune reaction becomes a threat to the body. Steroids have been used to decrease such hyperimmune responses. A few therapies were tried and their emergency-use authorization was granted to prevent a 'cytokine storm' and stop the immune system overreaction.

Tocilizumab, a monoclonal antibody that binds to an interleukin 6 (a cytokine) receptor, is one such immunosuppressant drug which is otherwise used to treat diseases like rheumatoid arthritis. Early studies from China suggested that patients who died with COVID-19 had high levels of this cytokine (IL-6) and tocilizumab could be useful to counter the cytokine storm. In COVID-19 response, this drug was granted emergency authorization for use in patients with moderate disease with progressively increasing oxygen requirements and in those on mechanical ventilation. Subsequent well-conducted studies, including one done by the pharmaceutical company which makes this drug, failed to conclusively show significant benefit of this drug. Many doctors felt that this drug had possibly a limited role and could be useful in only a small group of patients.[14] Again, like with antivirals, although we had initial studies suggesting benefit, subsequent well-conducted studies raised doubt on the use of tocilizumab. There are now some doubts about whether 'cytokine storms' really explain what happens in

---

[14] J.B. Parr, 'Time to Reassess Tocilizumab's Role in COVID-19 Pneumonia', *JAMA Internal Medicine*, 2020.

severe COVID-19, and whether we should be looking at other mechanisms, such as great damage to blood vessels or immune reactions to body components (auto-immunity) instead.

Convalescent Plasma Therapy

The fight against the virus is a story of experimentation and hope. Just when the evidence was ambiguous on HCQ and the data on other therapies was inconclusive, hope was pinned on the use of antibodies from the blood of people who had recovered from COVID-19. The approach was called convalescent plasma therapy (CPT). The approach of using filtered plasma from the blood of recovered flu patients has been used in the past. It was used in the Spanish Flu pandemic of 1918–19 and shown to save lives.[15] It was also tried in the treatment of polio and, more recently, in the Ebola epidemic. The rationale behind CPT has been that the plasma of recovered patients is expected to be rich with antibodies that can help COVID-19 patients fight illness effectively. However, we soon learned that all patients who recover do not necessarily have the same quantity of antibodies and testing the person's blood to see that sufficient antibodies are present became important before giving CPT.

---

[15] T.C. Luke, et al., 'Meta-analysis: convalescent blood products for Spanish influenza pneumonia: a future H5N1 treatment', *Annals of Internal Medicine*, 2006; 145(8):599–609. DOI:10.7326/0003-4819-145-8-200610170-00139.

Small initial trials suggested a benefit of CPT and this led to the need for larger good quality randomized control trials. Soon, research protocols for CPT were approved. While approval for CPT was given as investigational therapy, a few clinical trial sites for plasma therapy and plasma banks were set up in India. In the USA, plasma therapy was very widely used, without clinical trials. In India, in the absence of a specific treatment, CPT became very popular and family members started demanding plasma therapy. The lay public started thinking that this may be the magic bullet to cure COVID-19. The early analysis from ongoing trials on plasma therapy did not show much benefit.[16] Therefore, scientists have advised caution and stated that more data were needed to decide if CPT was useful and where it should be placed in the treatment of COVID-19. In October 2020, a randomized controlled trial of 464 patients from India was published in the *British Medical Journal* (*BMJ*), in which convalescent plasma was found not associated with a reduction in progression to severe COVID-19 and did not prevent death.[17] More studies are needed and are ongoing in other parts of the world. CPT may help some patients, but it may not be a game changer in the fight against COVID-19.

---

[16] L. Li, et al., 'Effect of Convalescent Plasma Therapy on Time to Clinical Improvement in Patients With Severe and Life-threatening COVID-19: A Randomized Clinical Trials', *JAMA*, 2020.

[17] A. Agarwal, et al., 'Convalescent plasma in the management of moderate COVID-19 in adults in India: open label phase II multicentre randomised controlled trial (PLACID Trial)', *BMJ*, 2020; 371 doi: https://doi.org/10.1136/bmj.m3939 (Published 22 October 2020). Accessed on 25 October 2020

Other Empirical Treatments for Complications

As we learnt more about the pathophysiology of COVID-19, it was realized that the disease is associated with increased clotting of the blood. Complications related to blood clotting were initially reported from China and the Netherlands. Other settings also started seeing these complications. Blood thinners (called anticoagulants) help in preventing the complications related to clotting in COVID-19 patients. These appear promising with empirical and early evidence. What is known is that SARS-CoV-2 invades cells in the lining of blood vessels. This results in the formation of clots. COVID-19 causes large clots to block main blood vessels, known as macro-thrombotic events. If this happens in the heart or brain, it can cause a stroke and other serious harm. The disease also causes small clots to form, known as microvascular thrombotic events, and if this happens in the lungs it causes a decrease in oxygen saturation. These small clots can also lead to local areas of bleeding.

Anticoagulants, which are commonly used for other conditions, such as heart disease, can slow the formation of clots. When these drugs should be used and whether they should be used in a preventive dose or a therapeutic dose is still unclear. Most hospitals now routinely use blood thinners in most sick patients admitted with COVID-19. In some hospitals, patients are at times also sent home on blood thinners due to the concern that clots may form at a later date. The utility of giving blood thinners is still unclear and is further being studied in trials.

Yet, There Has Been Success

One of the first drugs to have proved beneficial in a select subgroup of patients is the low-cost steroid dexamethasone. It reduces immune overreaction. This was the first drug shown to reduce COVID-19 mortality in the RECOVERY trial.[18] The use of this drug reduced deaths by one-third in patients on ventilators, and by one-fifth in patients on oxygen. It is less likely to help—and may even harm—patients who are at an earlier stage of COVID-19 infections. The evidence provided by the RECOVERY study changed the way many doctors were treating COVID-19. Previously, physicians were unsure about the utility of steroids as their use in the H1N1 pandemic (also known as swine flu) had shown conflicting results and suggested that its use may be associated with increased mortality. But H1N1 does not lead to the type of hyperimmune response seen with COVID-19. Therefore, there is definite benefit of using steroids in sick patients with COVID-19 infection.

Where Are We Heading in Terms of Therapies?

Nine months into the pandemic, there have been many clinical trials with relatively limited success. However, the mortality has been constantly declining. This can be partly attributed

---

[18] The RECOVERY Collaborative Group, 'Dexamethasone in Hospitalized Patients with COVID-19—Preliminary Report', *NEJM*, 17 July 2020. DOI: 10.1056/NEJMoa2021436.

to a better understanding of the disease and improvements in treatment protocols. We are constantly learning more about the virus and how it affects our body. Although we do not have a specific therapy, we have realized that some simple treatment strategies like supplemental oxygen, proning, steroids and judicious use of other medications does help in saving lives.

Many new paths are being explored. Like plasma, other antibody-based treatments are also being tried in clinical trials. Hyperimmune globulins, which have concentrated antibodies from convalescent plasma, and monoclonal antibodies, which are a single type of artificially produced antibodies, are also being looked at to boost immunity and fight COVID-19. Hyperimmune globulin can also be derived from animals like cows and horses. Animals are immunized with the COVID-19 virus spike protein and they produce high amounts of specific antibodies against the virus. These hyperimmune gobulins are processed and can be produced in large doses. Their utility in treating COVID-19 is being evaluated. Similarly, cocktails of monoclonal antibodies are being tried for prophylaxis and treatment of COVID-19 infection. We await the results of these ongoing trials, but there are some early disappointing results with trials in the USA being stopped for lack of effect.

HCQ is being used as prophylaxis, though its role in treatment outcome and mortality reduction has not been found and smaller trials have shown no preventive effect. Some data from India suggest that it provides some protection from infection and therefore it continues to be recommended as it is felt that it is a relatively safe drug. (Though the situation may change as more evidence emerges.) Most of the investigational therapies and repurposed drugs have not been found useful when tested scientifically so far and we are still waiting for a definite therapy. Yet, the way scientists, medical experts and researchers have worked together in solidarity to find a common solution has been remarkable.

Research, especially clinical research, has not been done widely or well in India. The pandemic is changing things. There is a new realization of the advantage and importance of investing in clinical and translational research. For India to be truly *atmanirbhar* (self-reliant), there has to be investment in research and frugal innovation. Science is making rapid advances and newer technologies and research are changing the way we practice medicine. The pandemic made us realize that to keep pace with advances in science and quickly develop new treatments, investment in research is essential.

For COVID-19, recovery is 98 per cent or more, even though it is recognized that there are lingering symptoms in 'Long COVID' patients. While effective therapies are awaited, treatment outcomes can be improved and mortality can be further reduced by ensuring timely care both by seeking care early and providing appropriate care. Hopefully, we will have effective and useful drugs and therapies soon.

Frequently Asked Questions

Is there any antibiotic available against COVID-19?

COVID-19 is caused by a virus of the family Coronaviridae. The medicines effective against viral diseases are called antivirals. There is currently no licensed medication, that is, antiviral to cure COVID-19. There is no proven antiviral against any of the viruses in the corona family. Antibiotics do not work against viruses (as the name suggests, these are effective against bacteria). For a COVID-19 infection, antibiotics are not recommended. However, a proportion of people affected with COVID-19 may also develop a secondary bacterial infection as a complication. In those cases, antibiotics may be prescribed by the treating physician. In any case, irrespective of the disease condition, antibiotics should be taken only on the prescription of a qualified provider.

Is there any medicine or drug which one should purchase in advance?

First of all, there is no proven drug available against COVID-19. Most are investigational, with evidence on their effectiveness being awaited. In any case, one should not store any medicine in advance. Anyone who needs medication for COVID-19 should be treated under the supervision of a doctor and, if required, in a hospital. You should have an adequate stock of cloth masks and hand sanitizers and must remember to use these whenever you go out.

Should I purchase a pulse oximeter in advance?

The pulse oximeter is used to measure the oxygen saturation in COVID-19 patients, especially those of mild to moderate severity. It is not needed for healthy individuals. In a home setting, the pulse oximeter would be needed only for patients in home isolation. In a number of states, governments are making a provision of supplying pulse oximeters for such cases under home isolation. If a patient is admitted in a facility, this would be available in that set-up. Healthy individuals have no reason to buy and keep a pulse oximeter at home, but any patient at home using a pulse oximeter must go to a facility immediately if oxygen saturation levels drop.

Are vitamin C or other food supplements helpful in the prevention or treatment of COVID-19?

Vitamin C is a known antioxidant with a role in controlling infections and promoting healing of the mucosal tissue. A healthy and balanced diet provides sufficient vitamin C. The rich sources of vitamin C are citrus fruits and vegetables. If we eat sufficient fruits, especially citrus fruits, we can meet our daily requirement. There is no scientific evidence to support that vitamin C or any other food supplements improve immunity or protect against COVID-19. People with a deficiency of vitamin C can increase their dietary intake of this vitamin.

Can vitamin D help in the prevention and treatment of COVID-19?

There is no proven scientific evidence on the benefit of vitamin D in COVID-19. Vitamin D is fat-soluble and is stored in the human body. Excess consumption and storage of vitamin D can actually be harmful. Studies in general do suggest that a low vitamin D level hampers immunity and many of us have low vitamin D levels. Therefore, one should avoid self-medication and people with a known deficiency of vitamin D should consult a doctor and follow their advice.

Are there any home remedies to treat COVID-19?

Home remedies and treatments have been widely used. However, these have not been recommended as standard treatment protocols. These may or may not be effective as most of these have not been tested under clinical trials. In India, many home remedies have been tried for centuries to strengthen immunity and protect against respiratory infections. The efficacy of these remedies is unclear.

What is the role of traditional medicine and therapies in COVID-19 treatment?

In every major disease and especially during a pandemic, there are always local treatments, practised in different parts of the world. These usually focus on good hygiene, improving immunity and enhancing well-being through the use of natural products and traditional practices. These approaches could be complementary, until evidence to support or refute the effects of the various immune boosters and therapies is available.

8

COVID-19 Vaccines: The Rays of Hope

When will a vaccine against COVID-19 be available? This has been one of the most commonly asked questions ever since the pandemic was declared in March 2020. After all, vaccines are one of the most cost-effective ways to prevent diseases, saving 2.5 to 3 million lives every year. Vaccines have helped in reducing the burden of several diseases, prevented deaths and even eradicated smallpox, one of the most deadly diseases on the planet. Children are protected from many diseases due to a robust immunization programme which is followed all over the world.

Most people know the story of Edward Jenner, considered the father of vaccination, who discovered the use of cowpox as a vaccine to protect against smallpox. However, vaccination or the process of inoculation was possibly practised for centuries in India and China. There are accounts of inoculation practice in eighteenth-century Bengal. It has been claimed that inoculation was a practice in India for thousands of years and has been mentioned in Sanskrit texts.[1]

The sequence of the virus was reported on 11 January 2020. The very next day, vaccine development efforts started. The first vaccines that were designed were RNA- and DNA-vaccines, and they were followed rapidly by viral vector-based vaccines, and others shortly after that. In just a few months, every available platform or way of making a vaccine was being employed to create a vaccine for SARS-CoV-2. In the ten months since the virus was first reported, over 300 candidate vaccines have been developed. More than fifty vaccine candidates have entered into human clinical trials, and a dozen have reached late-phase clinical testing.[2] In two countries that make vaccines, the regulators have given approval for early or limited use, but none has been licensed for full use as yet.

Since 1798, when the first vaccine was developed against the smallpox virus, there have been many, many vaccines developed, and every year millions of lives are saved.

In 2017, the *National Geographic* published an article on the US Library of Congress's ranking of ten inventions that changed history, and vaccines were listed at number five, behind the printing press and the light bulb, but ahead of refrigeration and the automobile. Preventing disease using the human immune system, instead of waiting for

---

[1] C. Lahariya, 'A Brief History of Vaccines & Vaccination in India', *Indian Journal of Medical Research*, 2014; 139:491-511. Available at https://www.ijmr.org.in/text.asp?2014/139/4/491/134094.

[2] Available at https://www.nytimes.com/interactive/2020/science/coronavirus-vaccine-tracker.html.

the disease to happen and then treating it or suffering its consequences, is a remarkable concept. The years 2011–20 marked the Decade of Vaccines, a commitment made by 194 member states of the WHO to an ambitious plan to ensure that all people everywhere lived free from vaccine-preventable diseases. While for children the vaccine coverage is now at 86 per cent, we have not utilized the full potential of vaccines for disease prevention, because we have not been able to reach everyone.

Routine immunization programmes for vaccination in childhood have been successful in reaching more children, thus saving people from disease and death, since the Expanded Programme on Immunization was initiated by the WHO in the 1970s. However, the potential for vaccines for epidemic disease remains underutilized. As described earlier in the book, when in 2013–14, the Ebola virus disease spread in West Africa, devastating Sierra Leone, Guinea and Liberia, a vaccine candidate was available, having been developed by the Public Health Agency of Canada, but it was not until nine months after the WHO declared the outbreak a Public Health Emergency of International Concern, that the world got its act together to use the vaccine.

It was the Ebola experience that led to the WHO's global Research and Development (R&D) Blueprint, which each year identifies the top ten threats to public health, and always includes Disease X, the unknown pathogen that will come from an unknown place at an unknown time. The experience also led to many international consultations, which resulted in the establishment of the Coalition for Epidemic Preparedness Innovations (CEPI), a grouping of state and non-state actors who are committed to the development of early-clinical-stage vaccines for outbreaks, which would address the issues of 'market failure'.[3]

The goal of CEPI, formally established in 2017 in Norway, was to make and keep ready vaccines that could be used quickly in outbreak situations for diseases on the WHO R&D Blueprint, and also to try to develop new technologies for a rapid response in case Disease X emerged. CEPI, supported initially by the governments of Norway, Germany and Japan, and by the philanthropic organizations the Wellcome Trust and the Bill and Melinda Gates Foundation, had India's department of biotechnology as a founding partner. CEPI had funded its first rapid response platforms in 2019, and in January 2020, it was able to fund the first three vaccine candidates.

Shortly thereafter, others, particularly multinational companies, with and without vaccine development experience, and governments followed with support for vaccine development at multiple scales, particularly in the US and Europe. The story of vaccine development during this

---

[3] Market failure refers to the idea that even though there is a need for certain types of vaccine, the companies that make vaccines are not interested in making them because they do not see any commercial viability in such products. In other words, if a disease affects the poor who cannot afford to pay for a vaccine, who will make it for them? Further, for an infectious disease outbreak, where the timing of the disease is unpredictable, the number of people needing to be vaccinated is unknown and if the disease occurs in a poorer part of the world, finding a company or group who will try to make a drug or preventive product like a vaccine is near impossible.

pandemic, while incomplete as of now, is a remarkable record of great speed, great science, solidarity among countries, and cooperation at a scale we have never seen before.

Nonetheless, while vaccines are awaited by some sections of society as the panacea to all ills, others have concerns that the speed may lead to compromises of ethics and safety. To know how vaccines are developed it is important to understand how vaccines work and the challenges faced in making them.

Why Do We Need a Vaccine?

We are infected every day by many pathogens. In most cases, we do not even notice, but with some infections, we become ill and mostly recover. Usually, the first time that we get infected is the worst experience of the infection, although with some infections such as dengue, the second infection may be worse than the first. During the first encounter with the pathogen, the immune system learns about the pathogen, recognizes its shape, particularly of certain proteins (and occasionally sugars), and creates an immune response. The adaptive immune response can be 'humoral', which effects its action through antibodies, or 'cellular', and this can take from one to four weeks to develop completely. The adaptive response results in the formation of memory cells which ensure that the next time the pathogen enters the body, the response is much quicker, and in many cases we may never even notice that our immune systems have prevented or restricted an infection.

While most infections can be successfully handled by the body—in the sense that very few of the many infections we encounter actually kill us—infectious diseases are not a pleasant experience. Repeated infections take a serious toll on health, and can affect nutrition and development. Vaccines which prevent infections or disease do what nature does, but they do it without making us ill. The advantages of a safe, predictable way of preventing infectious diseases are obvious.

How Do Vaccines Work?

Vaccines work in three steps: the first is to recognize the pathogen, the second is to make an adaptive immune response, usually in the form of antibodies which are produced by the immune system, and the third is to make a memory response to remember the infectious agent and how to fight it. Vaccines reduce the risk of disease by using the body's natural ability to fight infection by building a protective response ahead of time. Depending on the disease, vaccines can protect for years or even a lifetime.

A Quick Primer on the Immune System

Our surfaces have a number of ways to prevent bacteria and viruses from getting in, and these include the layers of skin and the mucus that line the mouth, nose, gut and lungs. Some pathogens make their way past these barriers by finding cracks or attaching to surfaces to prevent being washed away. When these pathogens enter areas that are supposed to be sterile, they encounter the first cells that defend all parts of the body against invaders. These cells are phagocytes ('eating cells') or macrophages ('big eaters'), which use harmful oxygen-based molecules to digest the invaders. Another class of phagocytes called dendritic cells (for their branched processes) eat the pathogens, but also break them up and keep pieces which they then show to other members of the immune system, the lymphocytes. The pieces that are shown are the antigens, usually fragments of protein molecules from the pathogen, which the lymphocytes recognize. The two kinds of lymphocytes are B-cells, which produce antibodies, and T-cells, which are of a few further types. The antibodies made by B-cells consist of one or more Y-shaped molecules, with the open arms of the Y able to recognize and interlock with the antigen. Once the antibody is bound to the antigen a number of things can happen: cells and/or destructive molecules are summoned which destroy the antigen, make holes in the pathogen or eat it up. B-cells receive messages from T-'helper' cells which recognize antigens to tell the appropriate B-cells what antibody to make. Each B-cell makes a completely unique antibody, so every day and all the time, new antibodies are made so that any pathogen can be handled. Antibodies mainly handle infectious agents when they are outside host cells, but when pathogens try to hide within host cells, they are sought out and destroyed by the 'killer' T-cells. A subset of T- and B-cells will become memory cells that will sit around and wait for the pathogen to come back, so that they can kill it quickly.

Why Does It Take So Long to Develop Vaccines?

Vaccine research and development is a long and meticulous process. From finding an antigen that may theoretically result in the human body producing a protective immune response to having a vaccine involves a series of steps in vaccine development that are increasingly complex, long, and expensive.

The first steps are in the laboratory to identify the antigens that are likely to result in a protective immune response. This can be based on the study of natural infections, animal models or information that comes from related pathogens—an approach that works for one virus may provide clues about how to approach another related virus. The preclinical studies in laboratories and on animals are followed by three phases of clinical trials on human beings.

The mumps vaccine is often considered the vaccine that was developed in the shortest period of time, four years. Before the COVID-19 pandemic, it was being considered that a vaccine against the Zika virus could be the fastest vaccine to be developed, because a Zika candidate vaccine went from concept to clinic in a few months, but after the disease subsided, many among the forty-five different vaccine development programmes have been stopped or delayed. On the other hand, in spite of years of research and more investment than in any other infectious disease, there are no proven vaccines against HIV. It took India nearly three decades to develop the first indigenous rotavirus vaccine since the identification of the virus strain. However, it seems that one or more of the COVID-19 vaccines will be developed and licensed faster than any vaccines so far, globally and in India.

The Various Phases of Clinical Trials

Clinical trials involve giving an experimental drug, vaccine, diagnostic test or management strategy molecule to assess the safety and efficacy of the intervention. Clinical trials are carefully designed and reviewed. If the clinical trial is for a new product, most countries require that all phases of testing are approved by a regulatory authority before they can begin, but in some countries, early stages of testing can be done without regulatory approval. Vaccine research can be grouped into two broad phases: preclinical and clinical.

Preclinical stage: This is the stage before human testing. Following laboratory experiments to design and characterizing the product that will be used as a vaccine, the candidate is tested in laboratory animals. In India, at least two small animals are used for toxicity testing, to see whether large doses of the candidate vaccine are safe. In India and elsewhere, depending on the vaccine, experiments in other animal species may also be requested, depending on how well the disease in humans can be seen in animals. The purpose of these studies is to show that the vaccines are safe. Sometimes, not always, immune responses are also studied in animals. When animal models of a disease are available, then the efficacy of vaccines in preventing infection and disease may also be tried. Preclinical toxicity studies are usually done in mice, rats or rabbits, whereas immunogenicity studies may be done in many other species as well, including guinea pigs, hamsters or ferrets. Animal models of a disease may be in any animal species listed so far, or in larger animals such as pigs or various species of non-human primates.

Preclinical studies usually take months if they are for a vaccine of an antigen or type that is already known, or years if done for a new vaccine. Failure rates are high—70 to 80 per cent of potential vaccine candidates identified in the laboratory never make it to the human testing stage.

Clinical stage: Human clinical trials are done in three phases, which are described in Box 7.2.

Box 7.2 Phases of Human Clinical Trials

- Phase I: This is done on a small number (around 20–40) of adult healthy human volunteers to assess its safety in humans beings. Participants are followed up for weeks, with safety being monitored intensively for the first few days and then less intensively for a period of days or weeks.

- Phase II: The researchers give the vaccine to a few hundred participants to assess safety in a larger number and measure immunogenicity. This stage is also used to decide what the dose should be. If the vaccine is to be used in a group other than adults, the vaccine is tested in the target group. Usually, the vaccine is compared with a placebo which does not have the active part of the vaccine. This stage of the trial will last a few weeks to several months, depending on how many doses of the vaccine need to be given, since the final immune

---

response can only be measured about a month after the last dose of the vaccine is given.

- Phase III: This phase is to test for efficacy of vaccines. The vaccine is administered to thousands (at times, tens of thousands) of people, with some given the vaccine and others the placebo or another vaccine. The goal is to make sure that there is no bias in who gets the vaccine and who does not. It is then observed whether they naturally encounter the pathogen, get infected and sick. The research team compares the two groups to see if the vaccinated people get less disease than the unvaccinated people, which indicates that the vaccine is working. The follow-up period is dependent on how common the disease for which the vaccine is made really is—the more common the disease the shorter the trial, but even with very large trials and common diseases, a phase III trial usually takes years.

Approval and post-marketing surveillance: After the successful completion of all the stages of clinical trials, when the vaccine is found to be safe and effective, the clinical findings are submitted to the national regulatory authority, along with very detailed information on where the vaccine is made and how it is tested at every stage of production. The regulatory authority examines the data and decides on the licensing. Even when the vaccine is licensed for public use and widely administered, manufacturers are required to collect and submit the safety data from the general public. This is often called post-marketing surveillance. It is also referred to as phase IV of vaccine trials, but phase IV trials can also be done by researchers for several reasons, including to measure how the vaccine is actually performing to prevent disease in the real world, in addition to continuing to collect safety information.

Monitoring Vaccine Safety

The safety of vaccines is very important because vaccines are given to healthy people. In addition to the safety data that is collected while the vaccine is being developed, once a vaccine is introduced into a national vaccination programme, safety data continue to be collected. Any unusual or above normal reporting of what has happened to people who received the vaccine is important. Most countries have a reporting structure so that any suspected vaccine-related safety events can be reported to public health authorities for a follow-up. The national adverse event following immunization system, or the national AEFI system as it is frequently called, is a tiered system in India, with reporting structures at district, state and national levels, and a committee that examines reported cases to decide whether or not the illness or condition that has been reported could have been caused by or is related to either the vaccine or to the vaccination process. This kind of system is important not only to study the relationship of a possible vaccine-related illness or injury, but also to monitor vaccine safety when vaccines are used in millions of doses as opposed to the thousands of doses in vaccine trials.

Any common vaccine safety–related features will be picked up in clinical testing, for example, fever, pain at the injection site, headache. Any condition that occurs in one in thousand or so vaccinated people can usually be identified, but establishing the relationship of a vaccine with a rarer event can be difficult. Any vaccine-related side effects which occur in about one in ten thousand participants are unlikely to be seen with any reliability in any phase of clinical trials, because the number of people participating is too few to pick up a strong safety signal.

What Are the Vaccines for SARS-CoV-2 Made Of?

The first vaccine ever made for smallpox used a living virus to induce immunity to a related virus. The idea of using a weakened virus or bacterium is one that has been repeated to produce many other vaccines like the BCG vaccine for tuberculosis or the measles vaccines. There are other approaches to vaccine development that have been listed in Box 7.3 and described in the following sections.

Box 7.3: Approaches for Vaccine Development

- Live attenuated vaccines: the whole living organisms, weakened in some way to not cause disease but induce an immune response.
- Inactivated vaccines: made of whole killed organisms.
- Subunit vaccines: parts of the organism that are important to induce the immune response, these may be purified from the whole organism, or could be made

separately as just proteins. These could have a simple structure or be complex, such as virus-like particles, which are virus shells.

- RNA vaccines: the gene sequence for a protein is coded on an RNA molecule.
- DNA vaccines: the gene sequence for a protein is coded on a DNA molecule.
- Viral-vectored vaccines: a virus acts as a carrier of the gene sequence for a protein.

COVID-19 Vaccines in Development and Related Platforms

Vaccines based on whole living SARS-CoV-2: Since the whole virus can cause disease, mutations are introduced to make sure that the virus becomes unable to cause disease but can still induce an immune response. Earlier, the making of these mutations was left to chance by repeatedly growing the pathogens outside their hosts, but now new molecular approaches make it possible to make many mutations very precisely. Two Indian companies, the Serum Institute of India and Indian Immunologicals, are developing SARS-CoV-2 vaccines using this approach.

Inactivated or killed whole virus vaccines: Viruses that cannot multiply cannot cause disease, so inactivating a virus, using chemicals like formalin can convert it into a safe immunogen. Because inactivated viruses do not multiply, we may need to use multiple doses of the vaccine and also give another substance to improve the immune response—this is called an adjuvant. The most common adjuvant is alum, which is also used in pickling and tanning of leather. Other adjuvants come from shark oil suspensions and can be harder to standardize. Many Chinese companies that have partial approval for their vaccines have developed inactivated vaccines, and the ICMR is working with Bharat Biotech on a vaccine that will enter phase III trials in November 2020.

Protein vaccines: A vaccine that consists of a whole or part of a protein is called a protein or subunit vaccine. Many subunit vaccines are produced in bacterial or fungal cells, so that large amounts of protein can be made easily. Many companies are working on protein vaccines based on the spike protein of SARS-CoV-2. Some, depending on the size of the protein, will need an adjuvant. Major multinational companies like Sanofi are developing a vaccine that will be made in armyworms, while other companies are trying plants. Because proteins can be floppy or change shape to forms that may not induce the right immune response, it is sometimes necessary to engineer proteins to stay in a shape that induces the best response. An example of this is the 'molecular clamp' technology which has been developed by the University of Queensland for the spike protein to keep it in shape before it sticks to the host cell. A related approach to protein vaccines is to make larger proteins that fold themselves to resemble whole virus particles. This approach of virus-like particles has been previously used for human papilloma virus vaccines.

RNA Vaccines: While there are vaccines on the market that use whole living or inactivated pathogens and proteins for prevention of infectious diseases in humans, there are no licensed RNA vaccines. Yet, RNA vaccines have a lot of advantages as a platform because they can be made rapidly and have fewer long-term safety concerns as they cannot enter the nucleus and leave the bloodstream quickly. To give the vaccine, the RNA carrying the sequence for the protein (spike protein for SARS-CoV-2 vaccines) is enclosed usually in a fatty nanoparticle. This resembles cell membranes and can deliver the RNA into the host cell where the messenger RNA is treated like it belongs. The cell uses its protein-producing machinery to read the message and make spike protein which is then released from the host cell and recognized by the immune system, triggering a response that results in both antibody production and cellular immunity. The first vaccine to reach clinical trial in March 2020 was the mRNA-1273 from Moderna, which is now in phase III trials. The first results for the efficacy of coronavirus vaccines are likely to come from the RNA or viral-vectored vaccines.

DNA vaccines: These vaccines resemble RNA vaccines in carrying the sequence for the gene codes for the protein that induces the right protective immune response, which is the spike protein for most SARS-CoV-2 vaccine candidates. But DNA candidates must enter the cell and then the nucleus to get the cell to make the messenger RNA. The messenger RNA will carry the sequence to where the protein is made. Getting the DNA into cells can be a challenge, and approaches include using electricity, or carrying the DNA on a plasmid to get the

DNA into immune cells in the skin or muscle. India's Zydus Cadila's vaccine uses the latter approach of a DNA plasmid. There are no licensed DNA vaccines for humans, but there are DNA vaccines for infectious diseases in salmon and horses and for cancer in dogs.

Viral-vectored vaccines: In infectious disease biology, a vector is an agent that delivers a pathogen, like mosquitoes transmitting malaria. Viral-vectored vaccines use viruses to carry the target antigen gene into cells. There are many such viral vectors, which have different advantages. The most widely known are the adenovirus vectors, which cause mild colds or asymptomatic infections in humans. The widely discussed University of Oxford vaccine, being developed with AstraZeneca and Serum Institute of India, uses a chimpanzee adenovirus with the SARS-CoV-2 spike protein. The chimpanzee adenovirus is used because humans will not have pre-existing antibodies to this adenovirus, while previous colds or infections may leave them with antibodies to the human adenoviruses, which could interfere with the vaccine. The Russian Gamaleya Research Institute vaccine uses two human adenoviruses, for the same reason of wanting to reduce any interference with the second dose. Although adenoviruses are non-replicating, meaning that the virus given in the vaccine does not multiply, viral-vectored vaccines can also be made using viruses capable of multiplying, like measles and pox viruses. Some vaccines are using weakened influenza viruses as vectors, so that a combination vaccine for both influenza and SARS-CoV-2 can be made.

How Is the COVID-19 Vaccine Research Being Accelerated?

Generally, it takes years to develop and license a vaccine. Many factors determine its success or failure. The long period and unpredictable outcomes, at times, discourage vaccine research. During a pandemic, a vaccine is needed quickly. A number of approaches have been used to speed up vaccine research and development.

- Rapid response platforms that use the information from virus sequence data to quickly design vaccines are being used. RNA and DNA vaccines may not have any licensed products for humans, but they have many years of development experience in humans. For viral vectors, two vaccines for Ebola were licensed in 2019 and 2020, showing that the platforms work.
- National regulatory authorities (Central Drugs Standard Control Organisation, or CDSCO, in India, Food and Drugs Administration in the US) have worked with global partners and industry to create regulatory pathways for the development and testing of vaccines. It is reassuring that the national regulatory authorities have clearly stated that patient safety will not be compromised; no shortcuts will be made for clinical evaluation. Instead, the agencies have put pressure on themselves by radically reducing the amount of time for the review of documents.
- Governments have funded large-scale efforts, instead of small piecemeal grants. Operation Warp Speed is probably the best-known global effort, but every

vaccine-manufacturing country including India has had government support for new vaccine development.

- Global cooperation and sharing have ramped up. In efforts coordinated by organizations like the WHO and CEPI, sharing of information and materials is being done at a level never seen before.
- Clinical trials for efficacy testing are being designed to be large and conducted simultaneously, so that results can be obtained quickly. This is also because potentially in some programmes such as Operation Warp Speed and the Solidarity 3 study, it might be possible to do head-to-head comparisons of vaccines.

Why Do We Need More than One Candidate?

The success rate at every stage of the preclinical and clinical trials is low. With regard to vaccines, out of every 100 vaccine candidates identified in an academic setting, only six will go on to become a vaccine. Therefore, the higher the number of vaccine candidates, the greater the chances of success.

Second, given the size of the world's population and the fact that no one manufacturer will be able to make enough vaccine to be able to supply to every country, it is important to have many manufacturers to ensure enough vaccines and buffer, in case some problem in making or shipping vaccines is encountered. Third, many manufacturers means competition, and competition of equally good products lowers the price, which is good for less well-resourced countries who need to buy vaccines.

COVID-19 Vaccines and India

India is the largest producer (by volume or number of doses) of vaccines in the world, and provides vaccines to UNICEF which then distributes them in Africa, South America and Asia. For UNICEF to buy the vaccines, the vaccines have to be pre-qualified or approved for purchase by the WHO. The WHO's approval process relies on the fact that the country which makes the vaccines has a national regulatory authority that meets the standards laid down by the WHO. India's CDSCO has met these criteria and ensures that the vaccines made in India are of high quality and safe. Indian vaccine manufacturers, which have grown in number and capacity since they were established decades ago, have good and long experience with manufacturing in high volumes. However, they have only recently begun modest investments in research towards new vaccines. With a population of 138 crore, India needs local and indigenous production of the COVID-19 vaccine to ensure widespread availability.

The development and availability of the vaccine in India has been part of some of the early discussions on the country's response to the COVID-19 pandemic. A national task force for vaccine research and development was set up in April 2020. The progress on the vaccines, both globally and in India, has been reviewed by high-level committees, and planning for delivery of the vaccines is ongoing. In early October 2020, the health minister announced a proposal to vaccinate 20 to 25 crore Indians by July 2021. In parallel with many such efforts around the world, discussions are on about the prioritization of target populations for initial vaccination.

Frequently Asked Questions

When can we expect the first vaccine against COVID-19?

Till October 2020, six vaccines had been given limited licence in China and Russia. While a definite timeline is difficult to predict, there is a possibility that some vaccines may be available by early 2021. However, vaccination will be an ongoing process and it will be two to three years before sufficient vaccines are available to vaccinate all those in need.

There are a number of vaccines in the last stage of clinical trials, why is it taking so much time?

It is true that there are COVID-19 vaccines in phase III of clinical trials across the world, with trials starting in India. However, there are no guaranteed successes, and we need to wait for the results to know what works and what does not. If successful, the data need to be submitted to the regulatory authorities for approval. This is followed by production by one or more vaccine companies and then supply, resulting finally in availability. All these steps are expected to take some time.

Who is likely to get the COVID-19 vaccine first?

The priority groups are likely to be health workers, who are in the frontline and who are required to interact with potentially infected people, the elderly and those with comorbidities who are at higher risk, as well as essential workers, which will vary from country to country.

The decisions are defined by the purpose for which the vaccine is used. If the goal is to prevent maximum deaths, vaccinating health workers and the elderly makes sense in the first phase. However, if the goal is to prevent transmission, then vaccinating younger people who interact more with others is the way to consider.

I am a healthy young adult with no underlying illness. When should I expect to get COVID-19 vaccine once available?

It is will depend upon the final strategy and how the population groups are prioritized. It is likely that first 20 per cent of the population vaccinated would have health workers, people in essential services and those with comorbidities and at high risk. In that case, a healthy adult is likely to receive vaccine at a later stage, likely in 2022.

What is vaccine nationalism? And how does the COVAX Facility work?

Vaccine nationalism is when a country ensures through buying vaccines in advance, or through ordering its own vaccine manufacturers to reserve doses for its own citizens, without consideration of how it may be preventing vulnerable people in other countries from getting vaccines. Many richer countries have done bilateral deals with companies that make vaccines to ensure that a certain number of doses are reserved for them.

To address the challenge posed by vaccine nationalism, the WHO has requested countries to participate in the COVAX Facility as part of the Access to COVID-19 Tools

Accelerator, as a cooperative purchasing mechanism. In the COVAX Facility, poorer countries which are or were eligible for support from Gavi, the Vaccine Alliance—which provides vaccines to low- and middle-income countries—will get deeply discounted prices or free vaccines, while richer countries will need to buy vaccines at a price in a pre-agreed range. For rich countries this will have advantages in that COVAX is negotiating with many vaccine manufacturers. With a range of products the chances of a vaccine being successful are higher, unlike with bilateral deals, where only that product if it succeeds will become available. Second, the prices negotiated as a group with larger numbers of doses will be less than for a single country's supply. The disadvantage is that the vaccines will come in tranches, so countries will get doses in batches depending on the size of their population, first for 3 per cent, then for 10 per cent, and so on. Many have argued that the approach of vaccine nationalism is not for global good, as no country is safe till every country and citizen in the world is protected from the disease. Even if a country vaccinates its own people, it will have to cut itself off from the rest of the world until everyone else gets vaccinated as well. Of course, these and other arguments have to take into consideration that no vaccine is likely to give 100 per cent protection from the disease.

What are 'human challenge trials' or controlled human infection model?

In phase III clinical trials, the efficacy of a vaccine can be assessed only when vaccinated and unvaccinated individuals are exposed to the pathogen. If the vaccine works, then vaccinated people will have less disease. However, natural infection is unpredictable, and it takes a lot of time for infections to happen and, consequently, for the efficacy of the vaccine to be measured.

In some situations for infectious diseases, human infection models have been developed where volunteers agree to be infected so that the disease can be studied in great detail. Although there has been a history of people being used as human guinea pigs and infected without treatment in the past, now human infection studies are very tightly controlled and monitored. Volunteers need to have a complete understanding of the processes, researchers need to be experienced and committed and backed by excellent facilities and clinicians to make sure the volunteers are looked after. The strain used for the infection is well studied, and ideally a good treatment for the disease is available. Human infection studies can be extended to test vaccines by first giving the vaccine and then 'challenging' the vaccinated volunteer with a known amount of infectious agent to see if the vaccine protects. This is an accepted methodology for many infections, and is required for malaria vaccine candidates where disease in animals does not provide good information about what happens in humans. Such trials would give quicker information about the vaccine, but are not a replacement for phase III trials. In mid-2020, the WHO developed ethical guidelines on the use of controlled human infection models in SARS-CoV-2 and had a discussion with multiple stakeholders, where about half of them thought such studies would be valuable while others had reservations. The UK has recently announced that it is planning to conduct human infection studies in the near future, with remdesivir as a treatment. It is likely that as with many other infectious diseases, we will gain valuable insights into the infection, in addition to potentially being able to test vaccines.

What is herd immunity? Do we really need COVID-19 vaccines or is herd immunity enough?

Herd immunity is also called herd effect, community immunity, population immunity or social immunity. It is a form of indirect protection from infectious disease which happens when a defined proportion of the population has been infected and has become immune to an infection. As an increasing number of people are infected or vaccinated, the number of people who can be infected ('susceptibles') decreases and transmission or spread also decreases. When herd immunity is reached, it is important to note that this is a feature that works at the population level—a decrease in spread within a defined group; it is not perfect protection of all uninfected people. At the individual level, the status of immunity depends on that person's exposure or vaccination status. This means that if a susceptible individual is no longer within the 'herd', then they are likely to be infected on exposure, and are not 'immune'.

When the level of infection or vaccination that is required is calculated, then the basic reproductive rate of the virus has to be known. The higher the reproductive rate, the greater the proportion of the herd that needs to be infected or vaccinated to prevent the spread. For measles, which is very infectious, we would like to reach 95 per cent vaccination to prevent outbreaks. At this time, data from sero-surveys in India shows 7 per cent seropositivity in a national survey at the end of August but pockets of high positivity in urban areas (56 per cent in some localities in Mumbai and 51 per cent in areas of Pune and 29 per cent in Delhi). This indicates that herd immunity is still far for most of the country, and we should be looking to a vaccine for more predictable development of immunity.

Antibodies are reported to drop quite quickly. Does a drop in the level of antibodies result in loss of immunity against the virus?

When the virus infects people, the immune system makes lots of antibodies directed against both the proteins that make up the shell of the virus, as well as other proteins that are made during the multiplication of the virus. The main antibodies that are measured are of two kinds—binding antibodies that stick to the viral proteins and neutralizing antibodies which stop the virus from infecting host cells. The binding antibodies are directed against different viral proteins, parts of the spike protein or the protein shell. Different tests measure different antibodies, so from the data available it is clear that there are differences in the decrease depending on which antibody is being measured. At present, there is no consensus and understanding on which antibody is protective and what the protective level of the antibody is. Even if antibodies do decrease, that does not mean that the person is necessarily unprotected, since there may be memory or T-cell responses which may be protective. To summarize, we need to wait and see what the data show—we have no clear answers now.

What if the vaccine is only 50 per cent effective? Will it be worth taking?

The COVID-19 vaccines under development now are first-generation vaccines. Regulatory agencies have stated that the vaccine should have a point estimate of 50 per cent efficacy; this means that the results of the trials should show prevention of at least half of the disease, but because of the size of the trials, it is possible that the actual efficacy of the vaccine may be higher or lower. Nonetheless, an imperfect vaccine will still protect a large proportion of people. Moreover, once a few vaccines are available, we can focus on improving their performance.

How long does immunity last after infection?

The duration of protection after infection is not known. Antibodies are usually a marker of protection, but it is feasible to be protected even when antibodies are not measurable, and it is possible to have antibodies that merely indicate that an infection had happened and do not protect. We want to know, but we need to wait and see what we find as we follow the people who have been infected. We need to see if they get the infection again, and if that results in disease or not. A small number of re-infections have been documented, but even among them most second infections were asymptomatic or mild. Again, for mucosal infections such as gut and respiratory ones, re-infections do happen, and very often, but they do not result in disease in most cases.

For how long will a vaccine give us protection?

The duration of protection after a vaccine can only be known only after the results of the clinical trials. It is too early to make any prediction about the duration of protection.

Do my earlier vaccinations have any protective effect against COVID-19 and can the vaccines available for other diseases prevent COVID-19?

There is some epidemiological evidence which shows that prior vaccination with BCG or measles may have some protective effects. However, this is mainly based on what is called ecological evidence, where results are noted based on populations and not individuals—this means that the evidence is weak. In Australia, India and the Americas, there are ongoing studies on vaccines containing BCG, recombinant BCG, polio and measles to see if they have any effect on preventing or modifying SARS-CoV-2, which will provide more evidence either way.

Do vaccines against pneumonia protect against SARS-CoV-2?

No. Vaccines against pneumonia, such as pneumococcal vaccine and haemophilus influenzae type B (Hib) vaccine do not provide protection against SARS-CoV-2. Although these vaccines are not effective against SARS-CoV-2, vaccination against other respiratory illnesses is highly recommended.

A vaccine against HIV/AIDS could not be developed after so many years. That is also a viral infection. Why should we be more hopeful about a COVID-19 vaccine?

HIV is a virus which infects and destroys immune cells, so it is very difficult to design a vaccine for HIV. Very few other viruses have immune cells as their primary site of infection, and in SARS-CoV-2 we know that this is not the case. It is important to highlight that a lot of the science that supports the development of new vaccine technologies, including many for SARS-CoV-2, actually came from the intense research and learnings from HIV.

Do immunity boosters help?

A good immune response depends on good nutrition and a healthy lifestyle. Dietary deficiencies, stress and poor sleep cycles are all known to affect immunity. Where deficiencies are identified, it makes sense to sort them out. Supplements and immunity boosters that are widely advertised do not have strong evidence that has been obtained by impartial, unbiased researchers. The best way to maintain good immunity is to eat in moderation, exercise regularly, stay connected to friends and family, and sleep well.

There are reports of change in the viral strains and re-infections in humans; does it mean vaccines may not be effective?

All RNA viruses mutate as they multiply. This is like a changed alphabet in spelling a word; for example, pediatric and paediatric are spelled differently but convey the same message. Coronaviruses actually mutate quite slowly for RNA viruses, because they have a proofreading mechanism. These mutations are useful for tracking the spread of strains between people and communities across the world, because we can sequence the viruses and see how the strains are linked to each other in time and space. However, most of these mutations have no effect on the critical functions of the virus, that is, to infect and to multiply. One particular mutation called the D614G mutation which appeared in February has spread around the world. This mutation, while allowing the virus to bind better to the ACE2 receptor, has no effect on the kind of disease in the host. It is also not expected to have any effect on whether vaccines work. There is also news about mutated viruses in minks in Denmark, but at this time, the mutations are unlikely to affect vaccination. However, with minks being infected so easily, we also need to track how easily the virus moves between animals and humans.

How long will it take for the pandemic to be over, after the vaccine is available?

A lot will depend on how well the vaccines work, how long the protection will last, and how many people we will be able to reach with the vaccines and by when. If we anticipate having vaccines in 2021 and then being able immunize most people in the world over the next two years, that brings us to the end of 2023, but it is likely that the efforts towards virus control will not need to be the same in later years as in the first twelve to eighteen months. Given what we are seeing with the asymptomatic infections, and the range of symptoms, it also seems likely that the virus may become endemic, perhaps like a more severe version of influenza. It is hard to have a firm timeline and prediction because we are still in the first year of the pandemic.

Disclaimer:

This information is based on current available evidence and is not medical advice.

Section IV

Getting Future-Ready

The 'triangle that moves the mountain' is a popular phrase in health policy circles in Thailand. The mountain here refers to any big or difficult problem. The triangle comprises knowledge, people's participation and political involvement. The people who coined this phrase probably believed that, with a coordination of these three, no huge problem is insurmountable.

In India's response to the COVID-19 pandemic, there have been many triangles working at different levels to move multiple mountains. These triangles are getting India ready for the future in order to enable the country to emerge out of the pandemic.

There have been three major stakeholders who have been working together and driving the response to the pandemic: policymakers (elected representatives and bureaucrats), health experts (public health as well as clinical medicine), and the community at large, that is, the people. It has been about collaboration, coordination and cooperation (another triangle) at various levels.

The battle against COVID-19 is likely to be a long one. It will probably continue at least until mid-2021 or the end of 2021, or even longer. This is assuming that most people are going to follow COVID-appropriate behaviours and one or more safe and effective vaccine/s will be available.

Also, battling the pandemic cannot be seen in isolation vis-à-vis a part of a country or even the country as a whole. The virus needs to be controlled in all parts of India and the world for the victory to be meaningful and lasting. The world has, in fact, become one small village, and the virus can travel quickly to any part of the world via someone who is infected but is asymptomatic or presymptomatic. This essentially implies that the response to the pandemic has to be sustained over a long period. There is no room for slack.

One of the ways to fight this long battle is to convert every challenge posed by the pandemic into an opportunity. We need to fight the immediate battles to win the war. We also need to keep learning and improving to ensure India's health system is prepared for the future.

9

Fighting until Victory: Public Health Response to the Pandemic

COVID-19 has taught us one important lesson. There isn't and will not be a success story till the virus has been addressed in every corner, from the smallest, remotest of villages to the largest, most accessible of cities, all over the world.

Over several months, we have witnessed how a few Indian cities and states, which were considered success stories because of the way they had handled the spread of the disease, soon started reporting a high number of cases. There have been two to three waves of COVID-19 cases in India. In October 2020, many countries across the world, especially in Europe, witnessed another spike, with the number of cases exceeding those during the first wave in March–April 2020.

The key to an effective response depends on how much we learn from each other—both from other countries and within our country. The pandemic has been a stark reminder of our interconnectedness.

The Proven Interventions We Know

The strategy is known. There are three broad buckets of interventions:

- **At individual and community levels:** Face masks and face covers; handwashing and respiratory hygiene; and physical (or social) distancing (together referred to as non-pharmacological interventions).
- **Public health interventions by the government:** Test (and isolate) and trace. Once a vaccine becomes available, that too becomes a public health/preventive intervention.
- **Treatment services:** Mostly through hospitals and other facilities set up specifically for COVID-19 patients.

All these interventions, and a few others,[1] need to be implemented in a suitable combination. A few more may emerge in due course of time.

The public health experts and task forces, at both Union and state levels, are already guiding the COVID-19 pandemic response in India. In this chapter, we list a few strategies and actions. Some of these are intended to reinforce what is already happening (and needs to be continued).

---

[1] The lockdown was a one-time intervention and there is near consensus that short-term lockdowns may not be very useful. However, there could be value in identifying hotspots and implementing localized containment and other interventions. Yet, going by the experience of the countries in Europe, which implemented a second lockdown in October–November 2020, it can be said that no strategy or intervention can be completely off the table.

A few other suggestions should be considered complementary to the ongoing initiatives. We hope that these suggestions will also help prepare policymakers and programme managers (at every level) to respond to future outbreaks, epidemics and pandemics.

The Fulcrums of Epidemic and Pandemic Response

Mount a knowledge- and evidence-based response: Epidemics and pandemics require a real-time response. One does not have the luxury to plan. Economist Jean Drèze has argued that 'evidence and understanding' are equally important.[2] While evidence has merit, the understanding one develops by experiencing ground realities is extremely valuable. We have witnessed during the pandemic that even as evidence was being generated, a lot could also be achieved by understanding and expertise. There are three broad tools to develop knowledge and understanding in the ongoing pandemic:

- *Public health expertise including disease modelling*: The response to pandemics depends on an understanding of the concepts of descriptive epidemiology: place, person and time. We need to ask: Where is the disease manifesting (place)? Who are getting affected (persons)? How is the disease evolving over a period (time)? Public health expertise is about asking questions and providing the answers with field-level understanding. The expertise

---

[2]   Available at ny/evidence-policy-and-politics.html.

is useful in scenarios with limited understanding and characterization of the disease conditions. Disease modelling could prove to be a useful tool as well. Stand-alone disease models may be of limited value; however, when combined with public health expertise, they can assist in planning for surge capacity and help assess the impact of interventions. Disease modelling can address knowledge gaps and equip us better to deal with the pandemic.

- *Expanded COVID-19 testing and the use of data for planning action*: Testing provides us with a fair idea of who are getting affected. It is essential to test as widely as possible to get a better understanding of the local infection pattern. The role of testing is far beyond the identification of cases. The testing (as well as treatment) data should be regularly collated, analysed and used for developing a better understanding of the disease pattern. This can be used for formulating action plans.

- *Scientific and epidemiological research*: Expert opinion-based response needs to be supplemented and at times replaced with more evidence-based and scientific response. As we go along, a lot of research in many spheres, including clinical science, basic science, as well as epidemiology, is providing and should continue to provide useful insights. The virus has taught us that as science evolves, we need to keep changing our strategy including testing and treatment.

With these three tools at hand, the implementation of interventions that are already known would be the key to success. When cases surged in Delhi in June 2020, it was better and effective implementation of the already known tools which brought the situation under control. Therein lies the proof that implementation makes all the difference.

Increase the breadth and depth of expert engagement: There is a need to engage a wide range of technical experts—public health specialists, epidemiologists, clinicians, microbiologists, data modellers, independent experts and communication specialists. The technical expert committees on COVID-19 need to be empowered with additional skills. The core committees and task forces need to be made more inclusive and functional at all levels, especially state and district.

One of the approaches has to be to go beyond formal expert groups and use all the 'expertise at large'. Many independent experts, researchers, think tanks and even newspapers have started analysing data, creating databases and sharing inputs voluntarily. These analyses have been hosted on dedicated websites, posted on various media platforms and published in newspapers. They have generated debates and discourses. This body of analysis and work needs more attention and should be approached in a systematic way. It is time that every available expertise is used. The voice of independent experts can be as powerful a guide as other knowledge that we have through systemic mechanisms. In the end, it is for the government to decide, but expert advice should be available for all. It should be free, fair and inclusive.

Actions Proposed at All Three Levels (National, State and District)

There are a number of interventions already being implemented to respond to the pandemic in India. We intend to assist policymakers and planners, at all three levels, to have a list of key areas which can benefit from their attention and intervention. The list below is not comprehensive (for instance, we have not listed vaccine deployment and administration, which is already being widely discussed). Similarly, a few challenges are likely to continue beyond the pandemic period (for instance, the need for an effective health information system or strengthening medical certification of the causes of death). These have been discussed in the next chapter.

Prepare well, develop surge capacity: Preparedness matters when responding to epidemics and pandemics. In India, we have witnessed that the states which have better functioning health systems and health services, and some past experience in such situations, responded far better to the pandemic, at least in the beginning. Across the world, the countries which had learnt from past outbreaks and epidemics were prepared and responded better. There is a need to develop 'surge capacity' down to the district level. Over the last two decades, there have been many outbreaks (SARS, H1N1, Ebola, Nipah, and so on), and these outbreaks have warned us that a pandemic of this nature is inevitable. There is a need, therefore, to invest in developing robust surveillance and surge capacity at all levels.

Risk communication and community engagement: This is an underused and underappreciated tool. Positive messaging is key to preventing panic and ensuring cooperation. However, that should not deter one from looking at and acting on facts. This will be essential for people adopting and continuing to follow COVID-appropriate behaviours. This will also go a long way in addressing stigma and discrimination. While national- and state-level interventions are important, districts should also focus on developing and deploying local strategies. It is important that people have access to authentic and reliable information on COVID-19. The success of non-pharmacological interventions is dependent on public participation and individual behaviour. Given the overwhelming evidence to show that people take risks, the relevance and importance of sustaining communication campaigns cannot be underlined enough. There is need for clear and transparent communication and the sharing of information on a regular basis.

Mobilize financial and human resources, in an equitable manner: The shortage of funds for the health sector is well known. For an effective pandemic response, both Union and state governments need to allocate, mobilize, optimize and prioritize funding for health. The pandemic can be used as an opportunity to address gaps and shortages in human resources at all levels and among various cadres. A few states have started the process. Bihar issued an order for the posting of nearly 5000 nurses. Rajasthan started the recruitment process for nearly 2000 community health officers. The Board of Governors of the Medical Council of India (the body which has now been replaced with the National Medical Commission in September 2020) recommended the posting of MD/MS students in district hospitals for three months. More such measures are needed. Clearly, just buying ventilators is not going to solve the problem. There is and will always be the need for sufficient trained staff to run the equipment.

Set up and strengthen public health laboratories till subdistrict levels: This pandemic has highlighted the urgent need to have well-equipped laboratories till the district level and public health laboratories till the subdistrict levels. These can start off as COVID-19 testing centres and slowly expand to include other laboratory services. These laboratories would contribute immensely to improving the disease surveillance system in India. In due course, the linkage of these public health laboratories with district surveillance units and epidemiology units will strengthen public health services.

Strengthen epidemiology units in every district of India: In the first week of April 2020, the Union government urged state governments to recruit and fill all vacancies of epidemiologists in every district in India. This has to be prioritized by the states, and if it does not happen now, it will probably be forgotten amidst competing priorities later. The government needs to have in-house expertise, supported by trained epidemiologists, at all three levels to fight the pandemic and be prepared to respond to all future outbreaks, epidemics and pandemics.

Improve data-recording and data-reporting systems for COVID-19: The pandemic should be used as an opportunity to improve the recording, reporting and analysis of disease data in the states and districts. There are many inequities being discussed, especially the effect of the pandemic on women, the marginalized population, and services catering to women and children. The health data segregated by various equity stratifiers should be analysed and used for action. It is an opportunity to consider making pandemic-related data available for analysis by independent experts to guide the process.

Enhance treatment services at all levels: In many states, a large proportion of the treatment services were being delivered through private-sector facilities. Creating and allocating COVID-19 beds in government health facilities is the only way to increase availability, affordability and accessibility of treatment services. It is an opportunity for the government to improve the provision of regular oxygen supply, ICUs, ventilators, and so on. Many primary health care centres in India need to have appropriate facilities to provide care to the patients needing admission, before their transfer to a facility can be arranged.

Focus on interventions and approaches to reduce deaths: There is a need to conduct clinical audits to understand the delays in admission and care of COVID-19 patients. Attention on improving the quality of services, facilitating access to health services, and developing special plans for mortality and morbidity reduction with a focus on high-risk populations will help. Reducing COVID-19 fatality rate would also require minimizing the delays (on the part of the patients) in seeking health care. Mortality reduction is dependent on both supply- as well as demand-side interventions.

Augment provision and availability of non-COVID-19 essential services: There have been reports about how the non-COVID-19 essential services were affected as resources and facilities were mobilized to respond to the pandemic. Immunization, tuberculosis treatment, and patients on long-term treatment for diabetes and hypertension experienced a setback due to the pandemic. These services need to be resumed and built up. This would be possible with directed attention and focus on these services.

Set up post-COVID clinics in every district of India: We need to monitor long-term morbidity associated with COVID-19. It is being increasingly recognized that even after recovering many patients still have post-COVID sequelae and they need regular medical attention and treatment. There is a need for post-COVID clinics to address the arising complications and examine patients for the impact of COVID-19 on other organs. While the initial post-COVID clinics are being opened at district-level facilities, to be accessible to people, these should be set up at the level of primary health care facilities. There is a need for proper training of physicians, and these clinics need to have adequate facility to provide the needed care.

A few additional interventions at the national level are listed in Box 9.1.

Box 9.1 Key Additional Actions at the National Level

- Develop a pool of national (including independent) experts and consider establishing mechanisms for all the states to seek their expertise.
- Document and share good practices and innovations from Indian states and various countries as well. Learnings from other countries and their experiences of handling diseases such as Ebola, SARS and Zika should also be explored.
- Consider expanding the 'national clinical rounds' to 'national epidemiology and public health rounds'.
- Support the centres of excellence developed in each state to provide training at the local level for optimum patient care.
- Start work and deliberations on how learnings from the COVID-19 pandemic experience can be used to strengthen overall health services.

Policy and Programmatic Interventions at the State Level

An effective response to the pandemic is dependent on the implementation of various strategies at the field level. Therefore, in addition to actions proposed at the national level, a few specific initiatives should be led by state governments.

- **Form an empowered and high-level group of experts at the state level:** Develop and implement regular expert review mechanisms of the pandemic response. The polio elimination programme in India had used such mechanisms very effectively and the experience and expertise of the people involved in those initiatives could be very useful, specifically in disease surveillance as well as in pandemic response as a whole.

- **Increase state-government funding and spending on public health services and infrastructure:** This is required for now and as well as for the future. Immediate funding is needed to rapidly strengthen testing capacity and public health laboratories across states.

- **Take a call on long-pending and much-awaited health policy decisions:** It is time that high-level political attention on health is used to take policy decisions such as setting up public health cadre and recruitment of health workers to fill all existing vacancies. It is also an opportunity to revisit the recruitment policies and salary issues, which are bottlenecks in filling vacancies and retaining health staff. Special legal measures should be taken to facilitate this process.

- **Revisit the health regulations and review the status of their implementation:** Effective use of regulations alongside sustained engagement with the private sector should be explored.

Proposed Interventions at the District Level

- A right mix of tailored, targeted and local measures with the use of data can effectively guide the response. The available expertise in the districts, including medical colleges, local development partners and their experts, and independent experts should be utilized.

- It is an opportunity to initiate multi-sectoral and multi-stakeholder collaboration for health at the district level. The coordination mechanisms for multiple agencies such as local municipal councils and corporations and the non-health departments should be initiated, if not already done, and then institutionalized to ensure better health for citizens, in the times ahead.

- Use this as an opportunity for gap analysis in health services at the district level. Get the staffing of healthcare workers right. This is an opportunity to fill all vacancies in the government healthcare facilities. The training needs of health staff at all levels in the districts should be identified and fresh trainings started.

- Prepare a district-specific response plan. Implementation challenges need to be addressed proactively and not reactively. It is likely that there could be fatigue among healthcare workers. This calls for plans and strategies to utilize the services of healthcare workers optimally. Regular, prompt and timely communication with the public is essential.

Box 9.2 The Talisman for COVID-19 and Related Public Health Interventions

In a pandemic response, the point to remember is that services are meant for every citizen. All of these services—

which includes preventive and promotive services, COVID-19 testing, treatment, hospital beds and even isolation beds—should be easily available, widely accessible and affordable for all. Any service needed for responding to the pandemic should be assessed on the parameters of AAA: accessibility, availability and affordability. This could be a talisman for the services to be provided during the pandemic. Whenever planning is being done at any level, important questions need to be asked: Are these services accessible to all people? Are these services (for instance, testing) available for all those who need it? Will these services be free and, if not, will people be able to afford the required services? The interventions should be continued till the answer is an unequivocal 'yes' at all levels. In fact, this talisman of AAA could be used for all health services in general.

A Powerful Tool to Make It All Work: Data-Based Monitoring

To ensure that strategies do not remain only on paper, there is a need to monitor progress based on local COVID-19 data. The polio elimination programme in India, implemented jointly in partnership between the Government of India and the WHO, has revealed the power of local-level data collection and analysis. The national polio surveillance project was instrumental in guiding and coordinating the response and eliminating polio from India. The experience and learnings during the pandemic will also be helpful when COVID-19 vaccines are available and need to be deployed. The district-level dashboard for various COVID-19 responses should be developed and used to the maximum potential. The public health and epidemiology expertise should be accessed from all possible and available sources to analyse and interpret this data for effective interventions.

Conclusion

The COVID-19 pandemic is not the first pandemic and it is not going to be the last. The fact is outbreaks, epidemics and pandemics are a part of our lives. The key is to keep learning from each of the challenges and use those learnings for future preparedness and response. India is still in the middle of the pandemic. We need to use the learnings till now to mount and implement an effective response at all levels till we win against the pandemic. It is possible and let us make it happen.

Frequently Asked Questions

Where are we headed in the fight against the COVID-19 pandemic?

One thing is clear: we will win against the pandemic. How and when is difficult to say as new understanding about the disease and the virus is emerging every day. The good news is that we can prevent the disease and control its spread by deploying the individual and public health tools at our disposal. We have succeeded in reducing the mortality associated with the disease. Once supplemented by additional tools such as vaccines, one hopes we can ride this through by late 2021 or early 2022.

I keep hearing a lot about surge capacity. What does it mean?

An epidemic or a pandemic, like the one we are experiencing, demands far more resources than usually available with any healthcare system. The ability of a healthcare system to ramp up additional resources to respond to an outbreak, epidemic or pandemic is called surge capacity. It involves planning for the worst-case scenario to employ the requisite healthcare staff and procure equipment (including medical devices) and supplies.

Is India better prepared for future epidemics and pandemics?

COVID-19 has been an entirely new experience with a new virus. It has given us an opportunity to be better prepared for the future. We have had experience in handling the 2009 H1N1 influenza pandemic in India. Though nowhere near the scale of COVID-19, the lessons from that pandemic, especially on vaccine deployment and administration, should prove useful. With the ongoing response to COVID-19, there is a better understanding of pandemics. There is also greater awareness about disease surveillance, public health testing services as well as epidemiology to prepare for future outbreaks, epidemics and pandemics. The learnings from this experience should and can be utilized for preparing India for effective epidemic and pandemic response.

10

Never Let a Crisis Go Waste: Strengthening Health Systems in India

India released the latest National Health Policy (NHP) in 2017. A year later, in 2018, the NITI Aayog released a five-year strategic plan (2018–22), which had four dedicated chapters on health. Both documents, especially the NHP 2017, identified the challenges in the Indian healthcare system. The government acknowledged issues such as low government funding for health, shortage of health workforce at all levels, focus on curative services, limited provision of preventive and promotive services, suboptimal functioning of the primary healthcare system, weak disease surveillance systems, and insufficient urban primary care systems, among others.

The NHP 2017 proposed increasing government spending on health to 2.5 per cent of the Gross Domestic Product (GDP) by year 2025 (from 1.15 per cent of GDP in 2013–14). The NHP also proposed that state government spending on health should be increased to 8 per cent of the state budget (it was around 5 per cent in 2015–16). It has been proposed to allocate two-thirds or more of the entire government funds on health for primary healthcare services. A public health management cadre has also been proposed. The NITI Aayog's five-year strategic agenda also made similar suggestions to achieve universal health coverage (UHC) and create a public health management cadre; foster development of human resources for health and strengthen the primary healthcare system in the country.

In 2018, India launched the Ayushman Bharat scheme (AB) to implement some of the policy proposals made in the NHP 2017. The AB is considered key for UHC in India, alongside the ongoing interventions under National Health Mission. The AB has two arms. One of them is the Health and Wellness Centre (HWC) that aims to strengthen and deliver comprehensive primary healthcare services in both rural and urban areas. This arm of AB proposes to upgrade 150,000 existing primary healthcare facilities to HWCs by December 2022. There is global evidence to suggest that nearly 80 per cent of health needs of the population can be met if the primary healthcare system is functional. The UK and many countries deliver health services through the primary healthcare system. While India has a vast network of rural primary healthcare facilities, the need for making these functional has been long recognized and articulated.

The second arm of the AB is the Pradhan Mantri Jan Arogya Yojana (PM-JAY).[1] PM-JAY aims to provide access to a range of secondary- and tertiary-level hospitalization-based

---

[1] PM-JAY is often confused with the Ayushman Bharat scheme, which actually is an umbrella name for both arms, namely the HWC and PM-JAY.

and admission-based services for the bottom 40 per cent of the population.

The Fifteenth Finance Commission had constituted a high-level health expert committee, which initially recommended increasing government funding for health to 2.1 per cent of the GDP. However, in the wake of the pandemic, it has been further revised to 2.5 per cent for health, to align it with the recommendation of the NHP 2017.

Learnings from the COVID-19 Pandemic

In early 2020, the health sector in India was about to shift gears from the policy formulation stage to the implementation stage. It is at this point that the pandemic happened. The importance of having a robust public health system has never been felt more acutely. We have learnt a few things in these nine months into the pandemic, which have been detailed in the section below and summarized in Box 10.1.

Well-functioning primary healthcare services as well as stronger public health services are essential to keep the society healthy: A majority of COVID-19 patients, nearly 80 per cent, needed only an initial interaction with health systems and no medical intervention during the entire period of recovery. They were either kept at CCCs, mainly to isolate them from healthy individuals, or were allowed home isolation. Such an approach reduced the risk of these patients transmitting the virus to others while visiting large facilities to seek care. Most of the interventions, be it contact tracing, testing, isolation or advising people on

COVID-19-appropriate behaviour, were being delivered by primary care and public health staff. It is for this reason that countries with a stronger primary healthcare system (such as Thailand and Vietnam) fared much better than countries with a hospital-centric health system. Taiwan largely controlled the pandemic through effective testing and contact-tracing approaches, delivered through the primary healthcare and public health teams.

Neighbourhood clinics play a bigger role in ensuring good health than large hospitals: The pandemic has shown us the utility of smaller facilities over mega hospitals. In the early period of the outbreak, big hospitals became overburdened as all suspected and sick people thronged them. Panic led even patients with mild illness to rush to these hospitals. This drove home the point that a good referral system helps in balancing out the load of patient care and ultimately leads to better patient care. During the period of the pandemic, a majority of COVID-19 and non-COVID-19 services were provided by the PHCs and neighbourhood clinics.

Health is about a broad range of services and providers: To stay healthy, we all need much more than hospitals and doctors. Health services are a combination of public health (preventive, promotive services) as well as medical care (clinical/curative services), among others. If it were not for preventive and promotive health services, which help in reducing disease, hospital services would never be enough to treat all the people who get sick. Also, health needs multi-sectoral inputs, and the importance of sanitation and infection-control measures have now become more evident. Focusing on only one type of service will not suffice.

Non-pharmacological interventions are equally important and effective: The war against COVID-19 has largely been fought by people adopting and adhering to the non-pharmacological interventions or 'the social vaccines' of wearing a face mask, handwashing, and physical distancing. Till (and even after) effective therapies or a few vaccines become available, these interventions will continue to play a key role in decreasing the disease burden. Other than for COVID-19, there are many non-pharmacological interventions that are proven against diseases such as diabetes and hypertension: healthy diet, regular physical activity, no smoking and moderate or no use of alcohol. It is time that the approach of encouraging people to adopt a healthy behaviour becomes mainstream for other health conditions as well.

Laboratory testing and diagnostic services are an important part of overall health service delivery: Testing can help in early identification of infection, prevent the spread of disease, and guide early interventions. This is also applicable for health services in non-emergency times. Testing forms the basis for other strategies which are planned at local and national levels and must be pursued aggressively.

Better functioning government-funded health systems are more effective in an early response to epidemics and pandemics: Pandemics are unprecedented challenges and no health system is fully prepared to respond to these without additional efforts. However, stronger health systems funded by governments mount a more effective response, which also allows for surge capacity.

Health services entail teamwork between health and non-health contributors: Keeping people safe and healthy requires interventions across a broad range of services, including testing for identification of those with infection, tracing the healthy who have been exposed and are at risk of falling sick, isolating those who are sick and can transmit infection, treatment for those who need medical care, and so on. For all of these, we need not only doctors and nurses, but also pharmacists, laboratory technicians and frontline workers. We also need coordination and collaboration with sanitation workers and community members. The pandemic has taught us that to tackle health issues comprehensively we need to move out of silos. Multi-sectoral collaboration is essential for comprehensive preventive and curative health.

Frontline workers are at the heart of health services: When the history of the fight against COVID-19 is documented, the efforts of frontline workers from the ASHAs, AWWs to ANMs will find a special mention. They are the ones who have guided the health system from the field and tracked the infection in the community. They perform yeomen services even during non-pandemic periods.

The health sector faces a paucity of essential supplies needed for delivering services: The shortage of PPE in the initial stage of the outbreak and, subsequently, a shortage of medical oxygen can be taken as indicative of supply issues in the health sector in India. Although the shortage was eventually addressed, this needs to be monitored on a regular basis. These shortages are indicative of an overall shortage of various types of supplies, such as medicines, diagnostic kits and other consumables.

The private sector has a role to play in health services which can be harnessed with effective regulation: In the early part of the pandemic, care was provided mainly by the public sector and since then, at every stage of the pandemic, the sector has played a major role. However, a proportion of COVID-19 hospital beds and ventilator-related services are being provided by the private sector as well. It is also contributing to COVID-19 testing services. But many state governments had to invoke regulations, including the capping of the price of testing and treatment services, to make these services affordable to a large majority of patients.

Health sector laws and regulations should be better implemented: It is telling that even during a pandemic the health system was exploited by some for personal gains and many items and services were sold at unacceptably high prices. Under conditions of severe stress on the health services, with supply unable to keep up with the demand, effective enforcement of health regulation becomes not only desirable but necessary. Legal provisions need to be invoked and health-related laws strictly enforced to do away with the black economy in medical supplies, ensuring hospital beds, testing services, masks and other essentials at affordable prices.

Health and economy are interlinked: The pandemic has affected the economy of nearly all countries, paralysing health and economic services alike. The link between health and economy for a nation came to the forefront during the pandemic. The economic impact was lower in the countries which had better and long-term sustained government investment in health services. Experts continue to emphasize that it is wise to invest in health and wiser to invest in primary healthcare and public health services. For a nation's economy to grow, investment in a good health system is essential.

There is a huge role of epidemiological, operational and scientific research in advancing health: In 2013, the WHO had published the World Health Report, which had highlighted the role of research for advancing UHC. When COVID-19 affected the world, everyone once again recognized the important role of various types of research (epidemiological, operational, clinical and basic sciences). The new research-based evidence empowered all of us to respond to the pandemic. It has brought focus on the role of researchers and scientists in the field of health. It is now time for governments to invest in healthcare research and support scientific work as well as scientists. The pandemic also highlighted how investment in translational research[2]

---

[2] Translational research is the process of applying knowledge from basic biology and clinical trials to techniques and tools that address critical medical needs.

is so essential. From making ventilators to vaccines, we have to have a good research and development system, and also promote entrepreneurship and start-ups in the health sector.

Health outcomes are dependent on collaboration and community participation: Collaborations among policymakers and technical experts, people and policymakers, among various agencies and many more have helped in dealing with the pandemic. Pandemic response is also about community engagement and participation in preventive and public health interventions. That is what we need for good health as well.

Box 10.1 Learnings from the COVID-19 Pandemic

- Primary healthcare services as well as stronger public health services are essential to keep society healthy.
- Health is about a broad range of services and providers.
- The neighbourhood clinic and PHCs can play a more significant role in better health than large hospitals.
- People adopting and adhering to preventive and promotive health interventions keeps the society healthy.
- Testing services are an important part of overall health service delivery.

- Better functioning, government-funded health systems are more effective in the early response to epidemics and pandemics.

- Health services entail teamwork between health and non-health contributors.

- Frontline workers are at the heart of health services.

- The health sector faced a paucity of essential supplies initially. These supply-related concerns need to be addressed.

- The private sector has a role to play in health services which can be harnessed with effective regulation.

- Health sector regulations should be better implemented.

- Health and economy are interlinked.

- There is a huge role of epidemiological, operational and scientific research in advancing health.

- Health outcomes are dependent upon collaboration and community participation.

An Opportunity to Strengthen India's Health System

The biggest immediate effect of the pandemic is that it has generated a greater public discourse on the need for stronger health systems and the health needs of the population. Never before had health issues received the kind of attention that they did in the wake of the pandemic. It laid bare the weakness of our healthcare systems and highlighted the challenges we faced. This awareness has already led to a few steps being taken to address the shortcomings, as detailed in section II of this book, with a few more listed in Box 10.2.

Box 10.2 Initiatives Already Undertaken to Respond to the Pandemic

- Teleconsultation guidelines were issued on 25 March 2020. These have the potential to make health services accessible in rural and remote areas.[3]
- Delivery of essential medicines at home was legalized on 26 March 2020.
- A toll-free national mental health service helpline was started in March 2020. The pandemic has brought attention on the need for expanded provision of mental health services.
- Practitioners of alternative medicine and Indian systems of medicine were allowed to deliver preventive and promotive health services. This has resulted in

---

[3] Medical consultations that can be done over phone or video call facility are termed teleconsultations. This makes consultation convenient and comfortable as well as time-saving for people. These could be especially useful for the elderly and those with chronic illness who just need follow-up advice. Teleconsultation will remove the inconvenience of visiting hospitals and reduce travel cost and the risk of getting infection while in hospital. Building up teleconsultation services will enable the government to provide access to health services in remote and underserved areas.

immediate increase of health workforce needed for the
delivery of public health services.

- The government announced a plan to set up public
  health laboratories to increase laboratory capacity as
  well as disease surveillance in India.

- Online platforms are increasingly being used across the
  country for capacity building of various health workers.
  Most of the trainings for the COVID-19 pandemic
  have been conducted through web-based platforms.

- The NDHM was announced on 15 August 2020.

Understanding the Health System

How does one define a health system? According to the
WHO, 'A health system consists of all organizations, people
and institutions producing actions whose primary intent is
to promote, restore, or maintain health.' A health system
comprises both public- and private-(formal and informal)
sector facilities and providers.

As one can notice in the definition above, health system
is a much broader and comprehensive concept. Yet, during
the pandemic much of the discourse on strengthening the
health system seems to have been focused on either adding
hospital beds or increasing human resources and some minor
upgrade in the infrastructure. This reflects an incomplete and
partial understanding of health systems.

A useful approach to understanding the health system
is to think of six functions, which sometimes are also
called 'inputs' to a health system. These six functions are:

(1) service delivery and provision; (2) infrastructure and human resources; (3) health financing; (4) medicines, diagnostics and vaccines; (5) health intelligence or information systems, and (6) governance and leadership.

The next question is why do we need health systems or what is their goal? Every system carries out the six functions (as above) to achieve a few final goals.

One of the key goals of a health system is to improve the health status of the population. This refers to improved health outcomes (reduced mortality rates, increased life expectancy etc.). The other dimension is reducing inequities, which means minimizing the differences in health outcomes seen in various population subgroupings (men–women, rich–poor, rural–urban, and so on) . This goal of the health system is very similar to the Indian concept of *sarve santu niramaya* or each person being healthy and without illness.

The other goal is to provide financial protection. It should work in a manner that health services are affordable to everyone. People who cannot afford them should get the services for free and for the remaining, the cost of procuring these services should not make them poor (remember, an estimated 40 to 60 million or 4 to 6 crore people fall into poverty due to health-related expenditure).[4]

The other goals include efficiency, that is, making sure that the resources are used in the best possible way to provide the maximum possible outcome; and responsiveness, in other words, meeting the non-medical needs of people when they avail

---

[4] The Government of India, National Health Policy 2017, the Ministry of Health and Family Welfare, Nirman Bhawan, New Delhi, 2017.

health services such as a clean waiting area, good behaviour from the medical staff, drinking water, clean washrooms, and so on.

A well-functioning health system is one which meets the goal it has set: keeping people healthy and treating those who fall sick in a timely manner. No one should delay seeking healthcare on account of cost or affordability. When these goals are not met, the health system is termed as a poorly functioning one.

The goals listed here can be achieved by identifying the weaknesses and challenges, and taking appropriate action. Initiatives and strategies that will help in achieving the final goals need to be worked out. The process of identifying the weaknesses and implementing interventions to tackle those challenges is termed health systems strengthening.

One related aspect is resilience. Resilient health systems are better prepared for additional challenges such as the management of disasters and epidemics, and are characterized by a strong surge capacity.

How to Leverage the Pandemic to Strengthen Health Systems in India

There has been evidence that stronger and better functioning health systems may not be able to fight the challenge from the beginning to the end, but they can surely handle the initial challenges, which gives time to policymakers and programme managers to develop surge capacity. The pandemic has brought the focus on the health system as a whole and the policymakers in Indian states are actively discussing about bolstering the health systems. We list here a few indicative suggestions for each of the six functions mentioned before:

SERVICE DELIVERY AND PROVISION

- **Make primary healthcare facilities functional:** The pandemic has given one unequivocal message: we need an effective and well-functioning primary healthcare system. There is piling evidence that a well-functioning primary healthcare system can tackle up to 80 per cent of health needs and can reduce the need for specialized health services. In a pandemic also, it was the primary healthcare system and services which was sufficient for 80 per cent of the health needs of the COVID-19 patients. Government spending on primary healthcare makes health services efficient, reduces cost and facilitates the provision of preventive, promotive and public health services.

- **Invest in and strengthen public health services and institutions:** The preventive and promotive health services are proven tools to keep society healthy. In the COVID-19 pandemic, it was the public health services which reduced the influx of sick patients into the hospitals. In a market-based system, these services are unlikely to be delivered by private healthcare providers. People depend on government facilities for public health services.

- **Strengthen urban primary healthcare services:** The population in urban India is nearly half of that in rural India. However, the number of urban primary healthcare facilities is about one-twentieth of similar facilities in rural areas. The primary healthcare system in urban areas needs urgent investment. This has the potential to decongest urban hospitals. Approaches and models such as community clinics should be explored and expanded.

- **Urgent and rapid expansion of mental health services:** There is an urgent and felt need to address mental health issues across India. There is a need for increasing government allocation for mental healthcare services. The provision of these services should be prioritized and scaled up. Alongside, innovative provisions such teleconsultations and a helpline on mental health issues need to be initiated. The mid- and community-level efforts to offer mental health services need to be explored.

- **Adopt innovative approaches for health service delivery:** These could include facilitating outreach services through medical colleges and increased use of telemedicine and teleconsultations for expanding coverage to underserved areas. The focus should be on establishing two-way effective and functional referral linkages. The services should be designed keeping in mind what people need (demand side), rather than what the government intends to deliver (supply side). There should be a clear linkage between the aspects of demand and supply.

INFRASTRUCTURE AND HUMAN RESOURCES

- **Make existing health facilities functional and set up additional PHCs as well:** Many more services could be delivered through the existing health facilities, provided the gaps in human resources and supplies are addressed. At every facility, the infrastructure, equipment and human resources should be available in the right mix to deliver services. Alongside (and not afterwards), additional facilities need to be set up to fill the shortage of the government primary healthcare infrastructure in India. More facilities need to be set up to meet existing population norms including the norms under the Indian Public Health Standards (IPHS). However, setting up facilities also means that human resources and other supplies need to be factored in. That is what would make the new facilities functional.

- **Revise the norm for UPHCs:** At present, India has a norm of one PHC for a population of 50,000 in urban areas. This is grossly inadequate to meet the needs of the urban population. In most countries, there is provision of one primary care facility for every 3,000 to 7,000 people. The shortage of urban primary healthcare facilities is one of the reasons that people go to nearest hospital for even basic needs. The bigger challenge is that since it is the primary healthcare system which provides a large part of public health and community outreach services, a weak system in urban settings also means poor provision of public health services. Whichever way we look at it, there is a need for rapid and accelerated expansion of UPHCs in all Indian cities.

- **Ensure sufficient and a right mix of the health workforce at every facility:** The health sector is a service sector and delivers services. Therefore, it needs people who have skills to deliver those services, including doctors, nurses, pharmacists, laboratory technicians and frontline workers. However, across several Indian states, the government health facilities are grossly understaffed, with vacancies in the range of 30 to 70 per cent. There is a need for public commitment and a time-bound road map to fill all existing vacancies in the health sector in India. An estimated 1.8 million trained people are needed in the health sector to address the shortage. Recruiting, retaining and retraining health staff is central to the functioning of health services and can contribute to employment generation as well.

- **Adopt a team-based approach to health service delivery:** There is an opportunity to develop team-based health services, not focused only on doctors. For example, for a diabetic and hypertensive patient who needs regular treatment, while a doctor can initiate diagnosis and treatment, aspects like monitoring blood pressure and sugar on repeat visits can be addressed by a nurse, who can dispense medicines as well. We need to empower nurses in government health facilities. This will also require public awareness and communication focused on sensitizing people about the roles of different healthcare providers.

HEALTH FINANCING

- **Develop and implement health financing policy interventions to make services affordable:** Affordability of health services is a key principle and financial protection is a goal of the health system. Health policies should be designed to ensure that people can avail health services without falling into poverty. This can be achieved through financial protection. There is global evidence that when any government increases their investment in health, services become affordable to people and they are financially protected. In the long run, the increased government expenditure on health reduces the overall healthcare cost, as the services become affordable and people start seeking early care and diseases , which would otherwise require expensive treatment, are prevented. In today's world, the health sector can be seen as a driver of the economy.

- **Both Union and state governments should increase funding in health in a time-bound manner:** Government spending on health is a social investment with high returns. There are global estimates that every rupee spent by the government on health gives a tenfold return to society. Healthy people contribute to the growth of the nation, by higher educational achievement, less absenteeism at work, and becoming part of a productive workforce. According to the National Health Accounts 2015–16, in India, the average spending on health per person per year is around Rs 4000; approximately Rs 1200 (30 per cent) of this comes from the government and around Rs 2400 (60 per cent) is borne by the patient (the balance by other sources). In many countries, the proportion of total health expenditure that people pay from their pocket, termed out-of-pocket expenditure, is less than 20 per cent (the lesser it is, the better it is for the people). In India, the union and state governments together spend approximately 1.2 per cent of the GDP on health. In many countries, this proportion is 3 to 5 per cent. In European countries, it is 8 to 10 per cent. India's NHP 2017 has made two related proposals: One, to increase government spending on health to

2.5 per cent of the GDP by 2025. Second, a policy recommendation that every state increase the allocation to health to 8 per cent of the state budget. It is time that both recommendations are implemented.

- **Invest two-thirds or more of government resources in primary healthcare:** The current expenditure on primary healthcare in India is around 50 per cent of the total expenditure on health. To achieve the proposed NHP target, government spending on primary healthcare needs to be increased. We have already discussed in earlier sections the importance and relevance of the primary healthcare system and public health services to keep the population healthy. Many services are best delivered and are cost-effective when provided through the primary healthcare system. The mental healthcare services and post-COVID-19 care services should also be delivered through the primary healthcare system.

MEDICINES, DIAGNOSTICS AND VACCINES

- **Increase the government funding allocation for free medicines and diagnostic schemes:** In India, for every hundred rupees spent on health, Rs 40 goes towards medicines and diagnostics. The government bears only Rs 4 of this share, that is, 10 per cent. It is not the cost of medicines and diagnostics during hospitalization alone but even the cost of medicines (unaffordable to many) that are used to treat health conditions such as diabetes and hypertension, which do not require immediate hospitalization. These medicines may be low-cost but they need to be taken regularly over a long period of time. This situation exists in spite of a number of state governments having schemes to provide free medicines and diagnostic facilities. Clearly, these schemes need to be rapidly scaled up. The government needs to explore innovative approaches that facilitate expansion of low-cost medicine stores as well as provision of free medicine from government facilities, even for those who get their consultations done in the private sector.

- **Ensure availability of essential medicines and diagnostics at all government facilities:** There are studies which have reported that assured provision of medicines and diagnostics results in increased patient attendance at a government healthcare facility. This in turn also makes health facilities and services efficient, as more people are benefitted at far lower marginal cost. Therefore, assured provision of medicines and diagnostics services should be prioritized.

- **Consider setting up medicine supply corporations, medical-parks and innovation hubs:** A few Indian states such as Tamil Nadu and Rajasthan have been able to reduce the cost of medicines and minimize stock-outs by setting up state-level medical supply corporations. A few states have created medical-parks with incentives to the private sector to set up the manufacturing units in the states. Such mechanisms should be actively considered to increase availability and reduce the cost of medicines and diagnostics.

- **Increase investment in research and development of vaccines and medicines:** India is considered the

pharmacy of the world. It produces a large number of
drugs used in many low- and middle-income countries.
India also produces and supplies safe and effective
vaccines, which are used in nearly two-thirds of the low-
and middle-income countries. There is a need for further
expansion of research and development in drugs, vaccines
and other areas. Initiatives need to be taken to ensure
increased availability of active pharmaceutical ingredients
in the country. Institutional mechanisms for capacity
building of health research have to be supported.

- **COVID-19 and other vaccines:** India has a large number
  of vaccine manufacturers and many of them are involved
  in COVID-19 vaccine research and development.
  Because of its manufacturing capacity, India's work on
  the COVID-19 vaccine will ensure equitable access to
  vaccines to the rest of the world. This attention should
  be used to increase government funding for investment
  in vaccine research and development.

HEALTH INTELLIGENCE AND INFORMATION SYSTEMS

- **Improve health data and information systems:** The
  health information system in India has a lot of scope for
  improvement. Updated information on aspects like status
  of functional beds, manpower, medical certification of
  causes of death are not easily available. Data reported
  by the administration, while not always complete, often
  provide information that is eighteen to twenty-four
  months old. This is rarely useful as even programme
  managers are aware that things would have changed since

then, for better or for worse. These indicate that a lot more is needed to have a robust health-data recording and reporting system. A well-functioning health information system can provide vital information to policymakers and programme managers to plan, develop and implement health interventions.

- **Establish public health laboratories and strengthen the disease surveillance system:** Indian states need functioning disease surveillance systems. They exist but need major revamping. Surveillance of SARI and ILI have been initiated and are supported by the laboratory network. The data generated from these channels should be regularly utilized to generate actionable information.

- **Build on the proposed NDHM as an opportunity:** The NDHM should be actively developed as the online platform for the future training of health workers and to monitor healthcare facilities. India's strength in information and technology should be leveraged for improved health information systems.

LEADERSHIP AND GOVERNANCE

- **Indian states to take the lead:** The impact of health initiatives is dependent on leadership and measures by state governments. State governments should consider conducting a detailed analysis of health system challenges and engage with experts to identify solutions. Thereafter, a time-bound road map for health system strengthening could be developed and launched by the highest level of leadership such as the chief minister of a state.

- **Set up public health cadre in all states:** Public health is the art and science of promoting, protecting and maintaining the health of people. Public health professionals focus on preventive and promotive health services and implementation of health programmes. A public health management cadre has been advocated in both the NHP 2017 and NITI Aayog's five-year strategic plan 2018–22. Each of the Indian states needs a dedicated public health cadre (at present, there are only a few who have one) and initiatives to deliver preventive and promotive health services.

- **Ensure effective enforcement of health regulations:** The role and importance of effective regulation in health services is widely known. Healthcare regulation, among many other actions, ensures that only qualified providers deliver services, that the health services are not overpriced, and helps to ensure that the quality standards are met. Health regulation came very handy during the COVID-19 pandemic in India. In mid-June 2020, when there were reports of excessive charges for hospital beds and laboratory testing, the government used regulations to cap the prices and make services affordable. There is a need to strengthen and enforce implementation of legislative and regulatory approaches in health across India. For example, the Clinical Establishments (Registration and Regulation) Act, 2010, has not been implemented by most Indian states.

- **Consider starting subdistrict-level health planning:** Indian districts have on an average 800 to 1000 villages or hamlets with total district population of 1.5 to 2 million

(15 to 20 lakh). In countries with efficient health systems, districts usually have 100,000 to 500,000 population, that is, the size of a block/tehsil in Indian districts. Health planning in India could be more effective if districts are subdivided into smaller units of 100 to 200 villages, for planning purposes. A formal mechanism should be considered to implement this across the country, and a few Indian states can take the lead. Every block can have a hospital, public health labs, and its own plan for health services (funding, human resources, equipment and supplies). It would be aligned with the idea of decentralized health planning in India.

- **Strengthen urban health governance and multi-sectoral collaboration:** The responsibility of primary care in urban areas was delegated to elected urban local bodies (ULBs) by the 74th Amendment in the Constitution of India. However, nearly three decades later, there is little clarity among the senior officials of different agencies on the role of that agency in providing health services. The urban primary healthcare services are relatively weak. Part of the reason is that while health is a state subject, in urban areas, primary care and public health are the responsibility of ULBs. Most ULBs do not have sufficient resources and do not spend enough on health. Of the total government health expenditure in India, only 4 per cent comes from ULBs. Of these, large local bodies such as Mumbai and Delhi have the lion's share of spending. The multiple agencies in urban settings need to work together for better health services.

- **Establish functional mechanisms for community participation and social accountability:** Most people do not know who is responsible for the delivery of specific types of health services. For example, in urban areas, it is the responsibility of ULBs such as corporations to deliver primary care and public health services. Hospitals are primarily the responsibility of state governments. In rural areas, services are the responsibility of state governments. The general public needs to be aware of who is responsible for the delivery of health services. This could work as an important social accountability mechanism.

- **Consider revising salary scales for all health staff:** A large majority of Indian states have salary scales that have not been revised for years. Low salary is the primary reason why people do not join government health services, and those who join leave soon thereafter. It is time states looked comprehensively at recruitment policies, and took the necessary steps to make government health services attractive enough to recruit and retain health staff.

These are some of the indicative ideas in each of the six health system functions. Our main purpose was to introduce a few ideas to policymakers and key decision makers.

First, health system strengthening is a more systematic and comprehensive process than tweaking one or two aspects.

Second, as one starts to implement such a process, it is worthwhile to conduct a thorough situation analysis of challenges in that setting, prioritize the interventions and prepare a detailed plan.

Third, it is important that the process is done with engagement of the highest level of health policymakers and other decision makers and is informed by advice from technical and subject experts.

Finally, all these interventions are done to ensure that the intermediate objectives of health systems such as access and quality are achieved. At the end of it, the final end goals are to ensure equitable health outcomes for all people, ensure financial protection, improve responsiveness and bring efficiency. It is not a one-time activity but a process that may take a few years.

We believe every single citizen (including the readers of this book) can play a role in strengthening the health system. For example, as a citizen one can ensure good health for all by highlighting health concerns to elected representatives and holding them accountable to the outcomes. Knowing and understanding various services and the need for a combination of services (medical care and public health) is important. This information can be used to generate awareness and influence policymakers. We believe that information in the earlier section has the potential to empower every reader, and they can use this information as per their role to contribute to the Indian health system.

India and the World Have Committed to Universal Health Coverage

In September 2015, at the United Nations General Assembly (UNGA), as part of Sustainable Development Goals (SDGs)

agenda 2030, all countries had agreed to achieve UHC. UHC
is one of the targets in SDG-3. India is a signatory to SDGs
and, therefore, has agreed to UHC. India further reiterated
that commitment by aligning the only goal of NHP 2017 to
the concept of UHC.

What Is UHC?

UHC by definition means that 'all people and communities
can use the promotive, preventive, curative, rehabilitative and
palliative health services they need, of sufficient quality to
be effective, while also ensuring that the use of these services
does not expose the user to financial hardship' (see Box 10.3).
At the heart of the concept of UHC are AAAQ: accessibility,
affordability, availability and quality.

Box 10.3 The Concept of Universal Health Coverage

The concept of UHC is often depicted with a cube, where
each dimension shows a coverage aspect, as follows:

1. **Population coverage:** All people need to have access to
   health services. (This dimension is about accessibility
   and equity.)
2. **Service coverage:** An entire range of preventive,
   promotive, curative, diagnostic and rehabilitative
   health services will need to be provided. In other words,

---

not just curative or treatment services but also services that will prevent diseases (or public health services) as well as testing and rehabilitation services. It clearly indicates that each of these services should meet agreed quality standards. (This dimension is about availability and quality.)

3. **Financial protection coverage:** Health services should be affordable for all—free for those who cannot afford to pay. No one should delay accessing services because of cost considerations. (This dimension is about affordabilty.)

UHC is a goal which all countries aim to achieve. Many countries have already made significant progress towards UHC which means health services are available, accessible and affordable to the majority in those countries. The goal of UHC can be achieved only through stronger health systems. Countries which have UHCs and robust health systems are also better prepared for epidemics and pandemics.

Conclusion

Before the COVID-19 pandemic, in the last two centuries, there have been two major pandemics. Nobel laureate Angus Deaton in his 2013 book *The Great Escape: Health, Wealth, and the Origins of Inequality* has analysed the cholera pandemic of the nineteenth century and then the flu pandemic of the twentieth century.[5] In his book, Deaton has argued that it was these communicable diseases that most European countries considered as a threat to economic development. Thereafter, these countries invested in developing public health systems. Much of the life expectancy and a lot of economic growth of Europe has come from its healthier population. COVID-19 is a similar global pandemic. It will be over after some time that is for sure. More important is how the pandemic and the post-pandemic period will be used to transform the healthcare system in India. That will determine the future of the health of the citizens. As an emerging economy and a modern country, India cannot afford to miss this opportunity. India has crossed the health policy formulation stage and is embarking on implementation. People look up to policymakers and health experts for the much-desired strengthening of the health system as India approaches seventy-five years of Independence.

Frequently Asked Questions

How many health systems does India have?

It depends on the prism through which we look and the political and geographical boundaries we draw. From the perspective of the national level, for international comparison, India as a nation has one health system. However, if we look

---

[5]   Angus Deaton, *The Great Escape: Health, Wealth, and the Origins of Inequality* (Princeton University Press, 2013).

at it from a more operational perspective, and because health is a state subject, India has as many health systems as its various states and Union Territories. If we look at it from the implementation perspective, each district can be considered a separate health system.

Is a health system only about hospitals and doctors?

No. The health workforce, doctors and nurses, are a part of the health system. The health system, as mentioned earlier, is a holistic concept in which we look at the entire process of inputs (which are grouped under six functions), intermediate objectives, and final goals.

Does the common citizen have a role in policymaking and health systems strengthening?

Citizen participation and community engagement are integral to well-functioning health systems and services. As early as 1978, the global public health community had identified community participation as one of the principles of the primary healthcare system. In the COVID-19 pandemic, we have witnessed the role of citizen participation in health services. More specifically, it is the citizens who, once empowered with knowledge about health issues, can contribute to an informed discourse and demand accountability from all stakeholders, and thereby also contribute to stronger health systems and services. People are at the centre of health services. They also need to understand their responsibility in preventive health.

What will achieving UHC mean to a common citizen in India?

UHC will enable every citizen, including the most underprivileged and marginalized person in the country, to gain access to quality health services without any difficulty. Let's take the example of a poor, old widow living in a remote tribal village of India. India achieving UHC would mean that she would have access to the desired health services within an acceptable distance and time frame. She will be able to select a health facility irrespective of her health problem, place of residence, or income level. She would have enough choice for providers, including for specialized care. She would not have to worry about the quality of licensed providers. She would have the assurance that the government has mechanisms in place for her to receive good-quality services and the confidence that she would be able to afford access to these services.

11

How to Stay Safe in the 'New Normal': A Road Map for Every Citizen

As you read this book, nearly everything (malls, restaurants, schools, colleges, Metro services) has either opened up or is in the process of doing so. Nothing, however, is what it used to be before March 2020. Will we ever be able to go back to our old routine and approach that we were once used to? If yes, by when? Is wearing a mask enough when travelling or should we wear a face shield as well? Do our urban local bodies need to modify public spaces to make the roads pedestrian- and social-distancing-friendly? Will cycles be the new mode of transport in urban India? Will work-from-home become the norm? No one has the answers to all of these questions, with any degree of certainty. The only thing that is certain is that COVID-19 will be around for a while. We don't know for how long but it will be some time before the 'normal' returns. There are many unknowns. There are evolving aspects of virus transmission. A lot needs to be done in terms of developing a 'new normal' for our day-to-day activities. We will need to evolve strategies that are practical and safe. We will have to take responsibility not only for ourselves but also for the vulnerable and high-risk populations around us, especially elderly people, children and those with comorbidities. In this chapter, we will look at how this new order will impact us at various levels: individual, community, professional space, public places and transport, and educational institutions, among others.

Adapting to Life with COVID-19

Things have already started to change in the way we deal with various aspects of life. Many offices and public places are adapting to a no-touch approach at the workplace. In many office and government buildings, taps in bathrooms have been replaced with foot taps or sensor-based taps to do away with the need to touch the faucet with our hands. Practices such as the use of face masks, checking of body temperature, and hand sanitization have become mandatory before entering most public buildings. Children are attending classes online and they have mastered the art. Many of us are delivering lectures, attending seminars and participating in social gatherings—virtually.

What is important is that we engage in COVID-appropriate behaviours (CABs) to stay safe and reduce the chances of transmission. We propose a 2-3-2-4 approach of CABs to stay safe.

The virus, the lockdowns and other social aspects of the disease have aggravated mental health challenges. Though mental health has always been part of the WHO's definition of health, it was seldom discussed. Moreover, mental health services have always been associated with some form of stigma. These services have also been insufficiently organized. It is hoped that mental health will now get the desired attention in policy formulation and programme implementation. In this chapter, we suggest a 1-2-3 or 'learn-to-connect-well' approach for good mental health.

In the period ahead, all of us have to return to many of the activities that we were accustomed to before the pandemic; how can we strike a balance of returning to those activities and reducing the possibility of getting infected with COVID-19? How do we protect loved ones at home, especially those who are at high risk? How do we return to work, schools and colleges and engage in daily activities such as eating out, going to the gym, visiting markets?

Staying Safe with COVID-19-Appropriate Behaviours (CABs): The 2-3-2-4 Approach

The onus on fighting the pandemic is on each and every individual. CABs are non-pharmacological interventions and other PHSM which individuals can follow to ensure protection. These are critical to win the fight against the deadly virus. These behaviours are based on evidence and listed and indicated in many official and government guidelines. For the sake of simplicity, we have clubbed these into four subgroups that list eleven action points which we call the 2-3-2-4 approach (see Box 11.1).

Box 11.1 The 2-3-2-4 Approach of COVID-Appropriate Behaviours

Physical distancing (2)	Face and respiratory hygiene (3)
Greet without physical contact	Wear face masks or covers in public places
Maintain physical distance	Avoid touching eyes, nose and mouth
	Maintain respiratory hygiene
Wash and sanitize (2)	**Responsible social practices (4)**
Wash and sanitize hands regularly	Educate yourself about COVID-19 and share only verified information
	Discourage crowding and avoid unnecessary travel
Sanitize and disinfect surfaces	Prevent stigma and discrimination
	Support others who may need help

Physical (or Social) Distancing Behaviours

Physical (or social) distancing has been the cornerstone for responding to the pandemic. It is a time-tested public health tool to prevent the spread of contagious diseases. The approach was adopted a hundred years ago during the Spanish Flu as well. Social distancing helps in reducing the transmission of the virus. We propose two appropriate behaviours regarding this:

- **Maintain physical distance:** We recommend maintaining a minimum distance of two *gaj* (six feet) at public places such as grocery stores, markets, dairy or milk stores, pharmacies, hospitals, offices, bus stops, queues, and any other public place. Physical distancing also needs to be followed when one is at the workplace and in a room/office with other people. Physical distancing should be followed with all other measures including the face mask. We need to be alert and maintain distance particularly with anyone coughing, sneezing or showing any signs of COVID-19. In a country like India, with its population density, maintaining physical distancing is a huge challenge and innovate solutions need to be found.

- **Greet without physical contact:** In India, as in many other countries, handshakes and hugs are common ways of greeting people. However, to tackle COVID-19 effectively, we have to make a conscious attempt to avoid physical contact while greeting. Namaste with a distance is safe and practical.

Face and Respiratory Hygiene Behaviours

Whether we notice it or not, we keep touching our face repeatedly—approximately fifteen to thirty times in an hour (yes, that is true). The virus can infect us through the nose and mouth. Therefore, every time we touch our face, it increases the chances of us getting infected. The risk can be reduced by three face hygiene behaviours.

- **Wear a face mask (or face cover) when in public spaces:** Using a face mask is necessary to limit the spread of infection. There is scientific evidence now that masks prevent the spread of disease and are a powerful tool in the fight against the COVID-19 pandemic. The mask should correctly worn and must cover both the nose and the mouth (more details in Box 11.2). Now that we know that an infected person could be asymptomatic and still transmit the virus, the relevance of masks has increased. Masks help protect those who wear it and those around him. Wear a mask every time you venture out of home. This is especially important for anyone with signs of cough, cold or flu, in which case, it is advisable to wear it even at home to protect family members. While a reusable, washable mask is good enough, those displaying symptoms of cough and cold need to wear three-ply surgical masks.

Box 11.2 How to Wear a Mask Correctly?

- Clean your hands before you wear a mask.
- Wear the mask in a way that the nasal clip is over the nose.
- External pleats should face downwards.
- The mask should cover the mouth and the nose all the time.
- If it is a mask with strings, tie upper strings first and then the lower strings. There should be no gap between the face and the mask.
- Do not touch the front side of the mask.
- Remove by first untying the lower strings and then the upper strings.

- Replace the mask after eight hours or when it is damp/humid.
- Do not reuse single-use masks.
- Dispose of the mask in the recommended manner (don't simply discard it on the street or floor).
- Clean hands after removing the mask.

- **Make a conscious effort to avoid touching your eyes, nose or mouth:** The mask is intended to serve as a barrier to touching the face. At the same time, we should be conscious of not touching our face after we have come into contact with open surfaces.
- **Maintain respiratory hygiene:** We need to cultivate the habit of covering our nose and mouth with a tissue or handkerchief when we cough or sneeze. This needs to be followed both within the home as well as outside. Coughing or sneezing into one's bent elbow is another approach. We also need to wash/sanitize our hands immediately after coughing or sneezing. This is a habit which can prevent other respiratory illnesses as well as the prevalent health conditions such as tuberculosis. Spitting in public places is a very common practice in some parts of our country. This needs to be stopped if respiratory infections are to be prevented.

Washing and Sanitizing

The virus spreads through droplets generated during speaking or coughing. It is transferred through hands which may touch an infected surface or object. Therefore, we need to get our hands and the surfaces around us free of the virus. One can follow these two methods:

- **Wash hands and sanitize regularly and thoroughly:** Washing with soap and water (any soap and clean water will do) for 20 to 40 seconds kills the virus. Alternatively, 70 per cent alcohol–based hand sanitizers can be used. The handwashing/sanitizing needs to be more rigorously followed when at work and other public places. Box 11.3 lists the steps to follow for proper sanitization of hands. There are many good quality videos available online to explain handwashing. Doctors and health workers keep doing this in their daily life at their workplace.
- **Regularly clean, sanitize, and disinfect frequently touched surfaces:** This renders surroundings safer. Sanitizing surfaces breaks the chain and complements handwashing. Household chemical disinfectants can be used for the purpose.

Box 11.3 How to Wash or Sanitize Hands Correctly?

- Apply sufficient amount of the sanitizer or soap in a cupped hand;
- Rub hands palm-to-palm;
- Right palm over left dorsum with interlaced fingers and then repeat the process on right dorsum;
- Palm-to-palm with fingers interlaced;

- Backs of fingers to opposing palms with fingers interlocked;
- Rotational rubbing of left thumb clasped in right palm and then repeat same step with the right thumb;
- Rotational rubbing, backward and forward, with the clasped fingers of right hand in the left palm. Repeat this process with the clasped fingers of left hand in the right palm.
- Once dry, your hands are safe.

Responsible Social Practices

In addition to the first three subgroups of behaviours, following a few social practices will contain the spread of the virus.

- **Discourage, minimize and avoid crowds:** As we know, crowds make it difficult to maintain physical distance and are often a fertile ground for the spread of infections. As such, social gatherings need to be avoided as much as possible. Also, it is a good idea to not venture out unless absolutely necessary.
- **Prevent stigma and discrimination:** In the initial days of the pandemic, there was a lot of discrimination against people who tested positive for COVID-19 as well as against frontline workers like doctors, nurses, police personnel and security guards. Stigma and discrimination adversely affect their mental health. Fighting stigma and discrimination is as important as fighting the virus.

- **Educate yourself about COVID-19 and share only verified information:** Studies have shown that people who had correct information and were well aware about various aspects of the virus had less stress, were better protected, and were coping well with the disease. As a responsible person, only seek information from reliable sources. Before forwarding social media posts, cross-check. Do not circulate or forward unverified and sensational social media posts. Wrong or unverified information can cause stress and mental health issues. There are a number of official websites of governments and leading international health organizations, which provide verified information.

- **Offer support to anyone who may need help:** The pandemic has impacted social, economic, mental and other aspects of individuals and families. How we behave during a pandemic is a reflection of our society as a whole. We need to show compassion and empathy, and reach out to anyone who needs help. This help could be in any form. Sometimes, just hearing out a person could go a long way in alleviating distress.

Social and Mental Health: The 1-2-3 Approach

How one copes with a pandemic such as COVID-19 depends on three factors: the individual, the community and the health system. Epidemics and pandemics have never been just medical events or crises. They have affected societies and nations in more ways than one. The mental health aspects of pandemics have been well documented. The key to combat them lies in not ignoring this vital fallout of a pandemic. It is important to take appropriate steps to improve mental health and seek support as and when needed. Positive mental health enables people to realize their potential, work productively, cope with stress and contribute to family and society. As part of good mental health, we also need to keep looking for symptoms of stress (see Box 11.4).

Box 11.4: Signs of Stress

- Excessive worry.
- Loss of appetite and fatigue.
- Helplessness and disruption of routine.
- Sleeplessness or difficulty in falling asleep.
- Suicidal thoughts or any other sign of depression.
- Irritability.
- Worsening of physical health such as increase in blood pressure or generalized body aches.
- Excessive fear of getting the disease and other signs of anxiety.
- Hoarding of sanitizers or masks or essential medicines.

Everyone is vulnerable. However, there are a few individuals who might be at higher risk than others. One of the approaches to having good mental health is to learn and read about the pandemic (only from reliable sources). Alongside, it is important to maintain basic hygiene and not become obsessive. Reducing exposure to television and social media could be helpful in reducing stress. Constantly engaging in conversation on this subject may increase stress and should be avoided.

It is widely known that mental and physical health are interlinked. While physical health can affect mental health, stress and mental health issues can reduce the body's ability to fight a disease.

Control what you can control is another approach to stay positive. Do not engage in depressive or negative discussions. Keep a problem-solving perspective. Think of a problem and then consider the solutions.

There is one message that should be communicated to one and all. Mental health issues are just like any other physical illness. Both physical and mental health issues are treatable.

Experts and government agencies, including leading mental health institutes of India, have come up with a few suggestions to address mental health issues. We have synthesized some of the common learnings in what we call the 1-2-3 (or Learn-Connect-Well) approach.

Three 'Wells': Eat, Sleep and Exercise

First 'Well'—eat well: A balanced diet, combining vegetables, whole grains, protein and fruits, is integral to our physical and mental health. It keeps one physically healthy as well as mentally agile. Everyone knows that overeating, irregular eating, or not eating enough is not good for health. Poor diet has negative effects on both the mind and the body. For example, overweight individuals may have lowered lung capacity and comorbidities which increase their chances of serious illness. Good nutrition is the key to a good immune system and works as an effective defence against COVID-19 and other illnesses. Eating well also includes the intake of fluids, that is, drinking water and non-carbonated drinks such as fresh juice, tea and soup to keep one hydrated. A good healthy diet will include three low-carbohydrate, high-protein meals per day with sufficient vegetables and fruits. We need to pay attention to what we are eating. Before eating, stop and think whether what you are going to eat is healthy or not. Make an informed choice.

Second 'Well'—sleep well: Sleep is important for good physical and mental health. It is as integral a part of our life as many other activities such as eating. Good sleep ensures harmony in our immune system. Sleep deprivation can lead to feelings of exhaustion, disrupting our daily activities, which may in turn cause stress.

Here are a few simple measures that may help a person sleep better:

- An adult on average needs seven to eight hours of sleep every day.
- Children need around ten hours of sleep every day.
- To ensure good sleep, maintain a regular sleep schedule. This can be made possible by sleeping and waking up at the same time every day.
- It is necessary (and helpful) to set not only a specific time to sleep but also, within a reasonable flexible window, one must have a schedule for work, meals and other activities.
- Regular physical activity and exercise also helps, for example, simple stretches at home, walking around the house, can improve sleep. Yoga and meditation are advisable.

- Eat dinner at least two hours before bedtime. Reducing or not having tea or coffee (or any other caffeinated drink) after evening also helps in getting better sleep.
- Reduce screen time. Avoid watching television or using the phone before going to sleep.
- Engage in conversation with family and friends. Spending time with children, family members, connecting with friends and colleagues helps bonding and good mental health.
- Reducing or preferably refraining from smoking and alcohol consumption would enhance quality sleep.

Third 'Well'—exercise well (and practise meditation): People who exercise regularly experience fewer mental health issues than those who do not. Physical activity is good for mental health as well as for the immune system. It helps reduce stress. The WHO recommends the following:

- Adults should engage in 150 minutes of moderate-intensity or 75 minutes of vigorous-intensity physical activity in a week.
- Children and adolescents should have 60 minutes or more of moderate- to vigorous-intensity physical activity every day.
- Elderly people with mobility issues can choose to have three days of physical activity a week to enhance balance and prevent falls.

Various institutes have indicated that yoga techniques—*dhyana* (meditation), *pranayama* (deep breathing) and *asana*s (postures)—can help to improve mental health. Meditating for around fifteen to twenty minutes every day can be combined with pranayama and asanas. Breathing exercises and pranayama have a positive effect on mental health.

Two 'Connects': Socially and with Nature

First 'Connect'—socially: It is important to stay connected with friends and family for good mental health. Social/physical distancing norms and restrictions on travel make this difficult but one can always find ways to connect while maintaining COVID-19-appropriate behaviour. Connecting socially is all about sharing, listening, being kind to people around.

As already mentioned, excessive screen time (in front of the television, computers, tablets and mobiles) as well as excessive use of social media can result in anxiety, stress and depression. Restricting and limiting social media and television/online time and replacing it with meaningful one-on-one engagement is a good idea.

Second 'Connect'—with nature: Connecting with nature is an integral part of keeping good mental health. There is evidence that spending time in the natural environment reduces depression and anxiety. When it is not possible to go out, even interacting with indoor plants has a positive impact. Spending time in the balcony or on the terrace can be helpful. Similarly, spending two to three hours every week in outdoor green spaces can be helpful. Create a small green area at home with potted plants. As the parks and public spaces are opening up, it would be worthwhile to go to these places when these are not crowded. It might be helpful to identify a time when the crowd is relatively less. Though things have opened up, it is important to continue to exercise caution.

One 'Learn': New Skills

The restrictive conditions many of us followed for several weeks and months indeed made life a bit monotonous. Even work-from-home can be very challenging, especially those who live alone or in a city where they do not have friends and family. (Now, many companies have allowed work-from-home for many months ahead.) It takes a toll on mental health. Working from home may save a lot of time spent on travelling. While this is good, it could be boring and challenging. This extra time at the disposal of individuals can be used in other productive activities such as learning new skills, which could boost one's confidence. The list of new skills one can learn could include anything from learning a new language to singing, cooking or craft making. Learning new skills can motivate you and that is a very good approach for mental health. Set yourself small achievable tasks for every day. Celebrate and enjoy those tasks and share with others.

Box 11.5 Face Masks: The Unofficial Emblem of the Pandemic Response

Face masks have become an unofficial emblem of the fight the against pandemic. These are scientifically proven in preventing the spread of infection. The masks are often being termed as the 'vaccine before a real vaccine'. In short, they are among the most powerful tools to fight the pandemic (as are handwashing and physical distancing). There are various types of masks available, which include the N95 masks, three-ply surgical or medical masks, and cloth masks.

In this box, we provide answers to key questions you may have about face masks and face covers.

Who should wear masks?

India has issued guidelines for universal use of face masks or face covers. As per current guidelines, everyone should wear a mask when going to a public place or outside homes. Follow government directives in your city and state. There is enough evidence to suggest that face masks reduce the risk of getting infections. Many countries have flattened the curve with the use of face mask in public places along with other measures. With scientific evidence that masks protect from disease, these should not be worn just because it has been made mandatory but because it is the right thing to do.

What are the guidelines and evidence on masks for children and adolescents?

Research indicates that children and adolescents are at as much at risk of being infected as adults. In July 2020, the WHO released guidelines advising everyone above the age of twelve years to wear masks while going out. Children between the ages of five and twelve years should wear masks as and when possible. Masks are not recommended for children younger than five years. However, appropriate protective measures such as face shield and reducing exposure are advised. This is an area of evolving understanding and the readers are advised to check for updated local guidelines.

Which is the most suitable mask?

There are different types of masks targeting specific populations. For health workers, N95 and surgical masks are recommended. Surgical or medical masks protect from large droplets. Home-made or cloth masks are recommended for the general public, especially those who are not in a healthcare setting. As the risk of transmission in public places is relatively lower than in hospital settings, cloth masks, providing a physical barrier and protection, suffice for the general population. However, if visiting a healthcare setting, it is preferable to use surgical masks. Cloth masks should be made of three layers and pleats. These three-layer cloth masks can provide protection from more than 90 per cent pathogens and bacteria. Effectiveness of all these masks depends on how they fit and how well the gap between the mask and the face is reduced. A well-fitted mask reduces the risk of transmission. One should carefully choose a mask but the broader principle is that anything that covers the face and nose is better than no cover. The masks should be worn properly.

When to wear cloth mask and when to wear a medical mask?

Healthy individuals, not diagnosed with COVID-19, can wear cloth and home-made masks. However, anyone who is symptomatic and waiting for test results or anyone who has been diagnosed with COVID-19 should wear three-ply medical (and surgical) masks. The following groups of people need to wear medical masks all the time:

- Health workers dealing with COVID-19 cases
- People who are sick and exhibiting symptoms of COVID-19
- Anyone taking care of a COVID-19 positive person at home

Why are masks with a valve not recommended?

N95 or other masks with a valve were designed to protect from air pollution. When a person breathes out, the valve in such masks opens, and the gases accumulated inside the mask go out. This also decreases the airway resistance as we breathe out and are usually more comfortable. This is useful for keeping one safe from poor air quality. However, if worn by a COVID-19 positive person, whether symptomatic or asymptomatic, it can spread the infection to other healthy persons as the air and the virus pass out on exhalation without being filtered. As we have learnt that an asymptomatic individual could have COVID-19, wearing such a mask with a valve can spread the infection. Therefore, the masks with a valve should not be used by the general public.

Should I wear masks while exercising or in the gym?

Face masks may reduce the ability to breathe comfortably and one can avoid wearing a mask while exercising. In addition, sweat can make the mask wet and make it difficult to breathe. The best approach in such a setting is to maintain physical distance.

Can someone develop oxygen deficiency or carbon dioxide excess due to the prolonged use of masks?

Medical/surgical masks can be uncomfortable especially when a person is not accustomed to wearing one. However, prolonged use of these masks, if properly worn, is not known to cause oxygen deficiency or lead to accumulation of carbon dioxide in the body. It is important that the mask fits properly and allows you to breathe normally. Do not reuse a disposable mask and always change it as soon as it gets damp.

Who should not wear a mask?

There are specific situations in which people should not wear a mask. These include children younger than two years old. People who have trouble breathing while wearing a mask or other specific respiratory condition, or people who cannot remove a mask without assistance, should not wear it. However, these situations and cases should be considered on case-to-case basis.

How to clean one's mask?

The single-use masks should not be reused. However, cloth masks should be washed regularly. It is advisable to wash masks separately from regular laundry. A soft washing soap or detergent can be used. It should be dried in proper sunlight, if possible.

Living in the Pandemic Period

How to stay safe and keep family members safe?

It is now necessary to accept the pandemic as part of our everyday lives till the pandemic is declared over. One of the things to be prepared for is the eventuality that a member of the family could test positive for COVID-19. What should one do when one has symptoms of COVID-19 or is exposed to someone who is COVID-19 positive?

A number of states have adopted the policy of testing on request. No prescription is needed and people can walk into any testing centre to get themselves tested. Government facilities offer testing free of cost. For people living in states where 'test on request' is not available, it is advisable to do a self-assessment of level of exposure and risk. It is important to take all the necessary precautions to prevent the infection from spreading. This could include self-quarantine for a few days and getting in touch with health services as soon as one develops any symptom. It may be worthwhile to think of a plan in case someone in the family needs to isolate himself or herself. Extra care needs to be taken for the elderly and for those with comorbidities. They should be encouraged to avoid unnecessary travel and contact, and adequate support should be provided for their care. The contacts of confirmed cases should get a test done. For contacts it is important to understand that the disease has an incubation period and they may not be positive on the first day. It is better to wait till the symptoms develop or when no symptoms develop, to get tested between the fifth and eighth day after exposure. The approach has to be self-care and ensuring that high-risk people are not exposed.

What are the likely outcomes if one is infected?

We now know that COVID-19 is a disease in which a proportion of people get infected but do not develop any symptoms (asymptomatic, around 30–40 per cent of the total infected cases). Then all those who develop symptoms are grouped into mild, moderate and severe cases. Each subgroup with COVID-19 infection needs a different approach.

Asymptomatic: A majority of COVID-19 cases are asymptomatic, which means the person will not have any symptom. In fact, the person may not know that he/she has been infected unless tested through molecular technique (in the initial two weeks) or for the presence of antibodies (through an antibody test), which develop after a week or two of infection. While being asymptomatic is good news for the individual, it is not necessarily so for the people around him/her. Evidence shows that a COVID-19 positive but asymptomatic person can be as infectious as someone with full-fledged symptoms.

Presymptomatic and symptomatic mild cases: A small proportion of cases would be presymptomatic, a stage before they develop symptoms. One can be infectious and spread the disease two to three days before developing symptoms. The majority of all symptomatic cases, nearly 80 per cent, would develop mild symptoms. People with mild disease would not need any specific treatment, except for the treatment of symptoms. For fever, antipyretic medicine is recommended; for cough, take measures to reduce cough. As for any COVID-19 positive patient, they need to work in the best interest of others to prevent spread and follow all CABs.

Symptomatic, moderate illness: People with symptomatic, moderate illness display more serious symptoms such as breathlessness and would have falling oxygen saturation levels.

They will need to be admitted and treated under medical supervision. This is the group which needs oxygen support. Unless their condition worsens, this group would not need ICU beds or ventilators. They recover with supportive care and specific treatment which may include steroids and anticoagulants.

Symptomatic with severe cases: A very small proportion, nearly 3–5 per cent of those tested COVID-19 positive, would need admission in ICUs and, possibly, ventilators or high-flow oxygen with a high-flow nasal cannula or a non-invasive ventilator to address the symptoms. Very few patients in this group may have a severe 'cytokine storm' and need aggressive therapy with anti-inflammatory drugs.

Home Isolation

Home isolation of mild or asymptomatic COVID-19 positive cases is slowly becoming an accepted approach. In Delhi, nearly half of all the COVID-19 cases were managed under home isolation. Many other Indian states have adopted this strategy. Home isolation reduces the burden on health services, while patients feel relaxed and comfortable in their homes and recover. Many individuals and families also prefer this approach to hospital admission. It is important that the family is aware of local and state guidelines to make home isolation a success. A few broad factors that we need to bear in mind:

- Isolation is a must for everyone who tests positive for COVID-19 and is either asymptomatic or has minor symptoms such as cough, headache, mild fever.

- A person in home isolation must stay indoors and in a dedicated room with an attached toilet. There should be enough rooms so that the infected person and other family members are well separated. If this is not possible, a better option is to be admitted in a CCC. Many states have these centres in hotels, which provide comfortable care and are attached to a hospital in case of any emergency.

- Select/identify a healthy caregiver who will bring food and other daily needs to the person. (Details in the next section.)

- For minor symptoms such as fever, cough and difficulty in breathing, seek medical attention, preferably through teleconsultations.

- Follow the 2-3-2-4 approach for CABs and 1-2-3 approach for good mental health. Monitor new symptoms. Know the signs and symptoms of danger so that you can contact health services (described earlier in this book).

- Collect and read official updated guidelines on home isolation.

- Check temperature and oxygen saturation regularly.

Home Isolation: Selecting the Right Attendant/Caregiver

People often have questions regarding who would be a good caregiver or attendant for a person in home isolation. A few broad principles for a family member as an attendant are listed here:

- The person should be in good physical health with no comorbidity.
- Preferably between twenty and fifty years of age.

- All principles of COVID-19-appropriate behaviour need to be followed by the caregiver/attendant. The person should wear a triple-layer medical mask when in the same room with the patient. Home-made or cloth mask is not recommended for the attendant. Even the patient needs to wear a medical mask.
- The attendant should avoid touching face, nose or mouth when in the immediate environment of a person in home isolation.
- Local authorities issue relevant guidelines for the attendant of patients in home isolation and those should be adhered to.

COVID-19-Safe Workplace

Measures such as physical distancing, handwashing, face masks, and sanitization are likely to continue till the pandemic is over. The 2-3-2-4 approach needs to be followed in order to maintain safety at the workplace. Thermal screening and provision of hand sanitizers at entry points have already been initiated at many offices and should be continued. However, it is important to standardize the thermal-screening device properly and make sure it gives accurate readings. In many places, they seem to be there more for visual comfort than for actual screening of temperature.

Alongside, the following are either already being enforced or should be implemented:

- Restructure office settings and workstations, ensuring physical distancing.

- Explore and set up physical barriers between people and workstations.
- Sanitize common spaces such as desks, meeting rooms and washrooms on a regular basis.
- Reduce physical touch points.
- Provide staggered working hours, lunchtimes and alternate shifts to reduce crowding. Offer sufficient flexibility to employees to work from home, as and when possible.
- Reduce gatherings in meeting rooms, conference rooms and boardrooms.
- Set up mechanisms for the sanitization of elevators and common places touched by many.
- Minimize visitors and shift to virtual meetings/interactions.
- Guidelines for visitors should also be defined; put signage and other markings for easy navigation.
- Special sessions (mostly virtual) are recommended for improving mental health (focused on yoga, meditation and other aspects). These can be extended to family members of the employees as well.
- Make sure the rooms are well ventilated and there is good cross-ventilation. If a central air conditioner is being used it should have fresh air coming in with adequate air exchanges.

These arrangements need to be planned by the management in consultation with employees. This will increase the likelihood of their implementation. The emotional well-being of the staff as well as their close family members should be actively promoted and encouraged.

COVID-19-Safe Educational Institutions

The seroprevalence surveys across Indian states and two nationwide surveys have found that the prevalence of antibodies in schoolgoing children is very similar to (and at times higher than) all other age groups. However, children do not have as many laboratory-confirmed cases and most of the infections are likely to be asymptomatic. There is emerging evidence that children are less likely to suffer from a serious version of the disease. But, studies have noted that young children who are asymptomatic have far higher viral load in their nasopharynx than older children and adults.

Continuing the education of children is of paramount importance. However, opening up schools is not only about protecting children but other family members as well.

By mid-October and early November 2020, schools and colleges in Indian states started opening up, in a staggered manner, where students in senior classes could attend school to meet teachers. A major concern in some families has been children attending schools and bringing the infection to other family members who could be at a higher risk.

As schools are and will be opening up, the approach has to be very carefully drafted and all standard precautions need to be taken. The Union and state governments have issued regular guidelines for schools, colleges and coaching centres. The broad principles would remain the same as listed for offices and other institutions. Temperature checks for everyone at the entry point, provision of adequate hand-wash and alcohol-based sanitizers and face masks need to be followed as per the guidelines at that point of time.

Attendance is unlikely to be mandatory for some time and a mix of offline and online/e-learning needs to be promoted.

Seating arrangements need to be altered and daily school assemblies need to be modified. Even the lunch break and designated areas for breaks need to be altered. Additional separators in open spaces and canteens with a high risk of infection have already been attempted in many schools. Bus and other school transport need to be reconsidered and redesigned.

Training and counselling sessions on mental health for students as well as staff should be conducted on a regular basis. It will be vital to develop regular (weekly or fortnightly) mechanisms for health education and knowledge sharing for COVID-19-appropriate behaviour. Special attention should be focused on reducing stigma and discrimination linked to COVID-19. Schoolchildren could be very useful messengers for CABs and should be regularly sensitized. They can take the messages on CABs to their families and help in preventing the disease. Many schools and colleges have explored a regular COVID-19 testing policy, but unless we have a good point of care test this will be difficult in most schools and colleges.

Safe Travel: In the City and Outside

Transport services have resumed, though with various restrictions. People have started returning to work. They use public transport, even though in a more limited manner than earlier. With Metro services resuming and buses and air travel opening up, discussions on travel-related safety are under way. Understandably, no environment is 100 per cent safe from the risk of infection.

New guidelines on public transport have already been announced by the government. More structural changes are planned. For example, the Indian Railways has come up with train coach prototypes to provide better hygiene and sanitation standards. There are plans to install foot-operated soap dispensers, fixtures with titanium dioxide (TiO2) coating that kills viruses, copper-coated handrails and plasma air equipment inside air conditioning (AC) ducts to sterilize and make the interiors particulate-matter resistant. There are plans to retrofit existing coaches with these amenities.

However, anyone who has had contact with someone else confirmed with COVID-19 should not travel. People at high risk should ideally avoid travel and, if they have to, should take special precautions and follow all the guidelines. Travel should be undertaken only when essential. These measures are likely to continue for some more time.

Accessing Health Services (Essential and Non-essential)

The fear of COVID-19 should not result in undue delay in seeking health services. This is important for non-COVID-19 essential services as well as for emergency services like acute cardiac events and strokes. This is also true for people suffering from respiratory illnesses with symptoms similar to COVID-19. Pregnant women and children too have special medical requirements which need to be addressed despite the limitations imposed by the pandemic. It requires action on both sides. The health systems need to increase and resume the services for non-COVID health needs. The primary healthcare facilities and smaller facilities, in particular, should be made functional and accessible. This would also reduce the risk of infection which may be slightly higher if people attend large hospitals, have to travel a long way and wait inside the hospitals.

Getting Back to Daily Life: Eating Out, Shopping, Going to the Gym and Jogging in the Park

For many months, people had minimized their outdoor activities and it has worked well until now. However, now people are getting restless and are eager to resume many activities which they have not indulged in for months and weeks. Restaurants, markets, malls and gyms are opening up as life returns to a semblance of normalcy. It is important to understand that the risk of infection is proportionate to the duration of potential exposure to the virus and to the viral load that one is exposed to. The need to take precautions cannot be overemphasized. For example, it is not advisable to work out with a mask on. Therefore, in addition to other precautions and guidelines, physical distancing is very important in gyms. Similarly, while jogging in the park, the best approach is to maintain a distance from fellow walkers and avoid sitting on the benches provided in the park. While lockdown has been lifted, and nearly everything has opened up, the virus is still around. We need to continue to take all the measures to reduce the transmission.

Handling Animals

There are limited indications that animals can transmit the disease to humans and spread COVID-19. The virus is spread through droplets produced when an infected person coughs, sneezes or speaks. It is advisable that people who are sick with COVID-19 and people who are at risk limit contact with others, both humans and animals. When dealing with animals, basic hygiene measures like handwashing after handling them or their food or supplies as well as avoiding kissing, cuddling or sharing food, are rigorously followed.

Conclusion

We are living in the period of a pandemic. These are unusual times which have affected our routine. However, as we face the challenge, we need to be prepared and respond. Staying healthy, taking good care of mental health, following known measures to prevent the spread of the virus, empowering ourselves with correct information will help us in fighting the pandemic and staying safe at home, offices and other public places. COVID-19 is a highly infectious disease but fortunately most people recover. The world is waiting for one or more safe and effective vaccines; as we wait for the vaccine, we need to keep following a few measures to protect ourselves and the people around us. That's how soon, together, we will win against the pandemic.

Frequently Asked Questions

How serious is COVID-19?

COVID-19 is a highly infectious disease. However, a large proportion of those infected or tested positive either do not develop any symptom or have mild or moderate symptoms. Nearly all people with mild to moderate symptoms recover with supportive care. It can be serious or severe for high-risk populations such as the elderly and those with pre-existing health conditions. However, it is difficult to predict who can develop severe disease. Therefore, everyone should follow preventive measures.

Who is at risk of developing severe illness?

This is not possible to assess with certainty. However, the elderly and anyone with pre-existing health conditions (such as high blood pressure, heart disease, lung disease, cancer or diabetes) appear to develop serious illness more often than others. There is emerging scientific evidence that people with comorbidities are up to twelve times at higher risk of death due to COVID-19 and up to six times more likely to be hospitalized. Men in all age groups are at higher risk than women. Clearly, reducing comorbidities and improving one's health is key to battling COVID-19. The experience of clinical settings in India indicates that people with two or more comorbidities in any combination, such as diabetes and kidney disease or hypertension and chronic lung disease, are at higher risk of serious diseases. In India, there are an estimated 55 million people with heart diseases and 70 million people with diabetes, which makes all of them high-risk.

In India, which age group and gender are more commonly affected by COVID-19 and who gets the severe/serious diseases?

In the first week of October 2020, a detailed analysis of data of around 200,000 hospitalized patients and 100,000

COVID-19 deaths was shared by the MoHFW.[1] It was found that 53 per cent of the total deaths had occurred among people older than sixty years. Another 35 per cent deaths were reported in people between forty-five to fifty-nine years of age. It was also reported that only 9 per cent of hospitalized cases were aged sixty or above. Nearly 62 per cent of all hospitalizations were less than forty years of age. Around 4.5 per cent of all hospitalized cases were children aged between zero to ten years. Clearly, the infection is lower among those who are young but it is not as though young people do not get ill. The analysis noted that the likelihood of death was higher when people had two or more comorbidities or underlying health conditions under treatment. At least 70 per cent of people who had died had a minimum of one comorbidity. Since many comorbidities in India occur at an early age (like diabetes), people of all ages are vulnerable.

Are men at higher risk in comparison to women and if yes, why?

The epidemiological data on COVID-19 cases from different parts of the world as well as India has shown that proportionately more men have tested positive for COVID-19 than women. Of all the COVID-19 deaths in India, 70 per cent of the deaths have been in men. This indicates that men are at a higher risk of suffering from moderate to severe

---

[1] Available at https://www.hindustantimes.com/india-news/62-5-hospitalised-covid-patients-under-age-of-40-govt-data/story-QEG3Id3xGirfuxUcBBEnXI.html.

disease. The reasons are not fully understood, and knowledge is evolving. Most likely, it is due to the way in which the immune system of men and women reacts. Researchers have found that in COVID-19, the immune response of men is mostly through cytokines and chemokine (the protective chemicals released by the immune system). The cytokine-based response, while being protective, can be harmful in excess, and results in severe disease, a phenomenon more commonly seen in men. In women, the immune response against COVID-19 is predominantly driven by T-cells. The T-cell-dependent response is more balanced and nuanced. There is more evidence emerging that oestrogen (a hormone in women) may have some protective role against the moderate to severe disease.

Can someone develop serious disease after getting infected from asymptomatic cases?

The people infected with SARS-CoV-2 who are otherwise healthy (asymptomatic cases) can pass on the virus to another. If that person is elderly, has weak immunity or underlying comorbidities, he or she can develop a serious infection. This is the reason that even people who appear healthy should wear a mask to prevent spreading the virus, as he or she may be an asymptomatic case.

Does COVID-19 affect only the lungs or other parts of the body as well?

There is emerging evidence that while COVID-19 is primarily a respiratory disease and affects the lungs, it can involve any organ of the body and can cause inflammation or direct infection in those organs. It has been found that the heart, blood vessels, kidney and other organs have also been affected. Neurological manifestations have also been reported. The disease can have a wide range of symptoms and very unusual and atypical presentations. It is clear that it is a multi-organ or a systemic disease.

What is the usual period in days for recovery from COVID-19?

Evidence is still emerging and we really don't know for sure. What is known that most mild cases usually recover within two weeks. Severe case may take longer, up to eight weeks. However, people may continue to show symptoms for a longer period and may require regular contact with health services (the long COVID).

What is 'long COVID'?

There are reports that many people who recover from COVID-19 continue to experience symptoms such as fatigue, body aches, chronic cough, tiredness, brain fog, etc. This is now being termed 'long-COVID' or 'post-COVID'. Most patients tend to recover with supportive treatment over six to eight weeks but a few develop significant and irreversible organ damage and they may need long-term support (like home oxygen or rehabilitative care). This situation demands that one follows up with such recovered people for specific complications on a long-term basis.

There is recent evidence that there could be a post-COVID-19 syndrome in children. How serious is this?

This is still being evaluated. It has been reported from multiple places in the USA and is seen in individuals who sort of recovered and then they have a fever, hyper-inflammatory syndrome which affects the skin, intestines, and also results in cardiac dysfunction. Many of these patients require ICU care to support blood pressure. This is a syndrome that has been called multisystem inflammatory syndrome in children (MIS-C) and a case definition has been developed. This is a new disease and knowledge is still evolving. It mimics another similar childhood disease known as the Kawasaki disease.

Can someone test positive after recovering from COVID-19?

There have been a few such reports from different parts of the world. Some people who have recovered clinically continue to harvest the virus in their upper respiratory tract for up to nearly three months. They can shed the virus as well. If tested again, they can be found positive, but after ten to fourteen days these are usually dead virus particles being excreted by the nasal mucosa and these individuals are non-infectious.

Can a person be reinfected with COVID-19?

There are not many reports that we can classically categorize under reinfection as of now. To classify any case as reinfection, the genomic sequence of the virus from both episodes should be conducted. There have been only a few such cases of reinfections verified based on genomic sequence out of the 45 million cases reported till the end of October 2020. Based on this information, it is too early to make any conclusive reference. As the pandemic progresses and more and more people recover we may come to know how much of a problem reinfection is.

Does air pollution increase the chance of COVID-19 infection?

There have been studies which have indicated that increased air pollution or PM2.5 level is associated with increase in the morbidity and mortality by 10–17 per cent.[2] Pollution causes airway inflammation and predisposes one to infection. More specifically, increase in air pollution results in higher number of cases of chronic respiratory and cardiac diseases such as asthma and chronic bronchitis. These conditions already burden the respiratory and cardiac system of an individual. Thereafter, if a person get COVID-19 infection, it is likely that the already burdened immune system and the inflammation caused by pollution in the system of that individual may not be able to fully handle the disease. Therefore, air pollution is likely to affect the moderate to severe cases of the disease. Studies have reported that the mitigation of air pollution can reduce COVID-19 mortality but can also help in reducing the future mortality.

---

[2] Available at https://www.sciencedirect.com/science/article/pii/S0301054620301099.

How can winter affect COVID-19 infections?

It is widely known that in most countries respiratory illnesses as well as infections due to seasonal flu viruses increase in the winter months. India's flu season has been shown to have two peaks, in the monsoon and the winter months. The available evidence shows that the peak in winters is just half of what is seen during the monsoon. The possible reasons include that (a) the viruses survive longer in the environment in cold temperature; (b) people tend to stay indoors during winter and result in crowding together in non-ventilated rooms. Winter is a festive season as well as a holiday season in India. During these months, people usually gather for family meetings, markets are crowded, and people might already have common cold and other seasonal infections. All these conditions are favourable for COVID-19 to spread. The government has already advised people to avoid gatherings and reduce unnecessary visits to markets in winters and afterwards. The best approach to adopt is to keep following the government advisory and guidelines on these aspects. Thus, while there is a probability of increased transmission, if people adhere to CABs, the situation can be controlled.

In many countries, cases of influenza are lower than all the previous years: why?

The countries which have good disease surveillance or reporting systems have noted a decline in influenza cases during the year. Experts have considered and explored many possible reasons for this. One possible explanation is that the public health and social measures being implemented for COVID-19 have contributed to reduced influenza cases. Physical distancing and masks have the potential to reduce many respiratory infections including tuberculosis. There are some other hypotheses and early work on those is being done. These include exploring the potential role of flu vaccine in reducing the chance of COVID-19 transmission, although this seems unlikely. However, things are at an early stage.

Are there differences between the symptoms caused by the seasonal flu and COVID-19?

There are many common symptoms between seasonal flu and COVID-19. There are a few broad principles, which can be followed to differentiate between these two as well as other respiratory illnesses. Cough and cold could mean an allergy. Fever with cough and cold is a symptom of the flu, if it is flu season. When an individual has fever with a cough which is complicated by breathlessness, these could be symptoms of a COVID-19 infection. There is a lot of overlap among the symptoms of other respiratory viral infections and COVID-19, and testing to rule out COVID-19 should be done in anyone with flu-like symptoms during the pandemic. These are also commonly called ILI. If symptoms progress to breathing difficulty along with other respiratory symptoms they are named SARI. Therefore, it is advised that whenever in doubt, especially when COVID-19 cases are being reported from your area, get tested.

I keep hearing about mutation in SARS-CoV-2. What does it mean for the severity of disease?

The mutation is a minor change in viral genomic sequence. All viruses mutate which helps them to adapt to continue to infect the human host. SARS-CoV-2 is fairly stable, yet there have been around 15,000 mutations which have been reported till September 2020. But most of these mutations have been in non-significant section of the viruses. There is no evidence that mutations in the various parts of SARS-CoV-2 would alter its ability to cause disease. Current evidence also does not suggest that any significant mutation has occurred to make the vaccines being developed ineffective.

What is the probability of a confirmed COVID-19 case transmitting the virus to contacts?

A study published in the journal *Science* towards the end of September 2020[3] noted that nearly seven out of every ten confirmed cases did not pass on the infection to anyone, even to their family members. However, a small proportion of confirmed cases, around 1 per cent, resulted in five to forty new infections. A key takeaway from this study is that while one needs to follow precautions and public health and social measures, there is no need to panic if one comes in contact with a COVID-19 case. If precautions are taken, the possibility of the transmission of the virus is reduced.

---

[3] R. Laxminarayan, et al., *Science*, 2020; 10.1126/science.abd7672.

What do we know about the risk of transmission from a confined space?

The study in the journal *Science*[4] had found that people using long-distance or long-duration shared transport had a high risk of transmission. In fact, this risk was found to be higher than the risk of transmission to those living in the same household. These findings have implications on the use of long-distance mode of travel such as buses and trains.

Which COVID-19 test should one get done?

There are two broad types of COVID-19 tests: antigen and antibody tests. Antigen tests such as RT-PCR and RAT are conducted to identify current COVID-19 infection, to detect whether a person is infected or not. Therefore, if one has symptoms or is suspected to have developed COVID-19, then antigen tests should be done. The antibody tests are to detect past infections. If one wants to check if he or she has been infected with COVID-19 in the past (such as asymptomatic infection), then the antibody test is done. In a sero-survey conducted to detect the level of past infection in the population as well, antibody tests are conducted.

How likely is anyone in the community to catch COVID-19?

The risk depends on the spread of infection in the setting and the risk behaviour adopted by the people. If one follows standard CAB, the risk is minimized.

---

[4] Ibid.

Are there things I should not do to protect myself from COVID-19?

The key is to follow CABs at all times. A few harmful behaviours like the following should ideally be avoided:

- Smoking (it is the best time to quit smoking).
- Wearing multiple masks (handling of these masks can be challenging and put you at additional risk).
- Taking antibiotics (this is a viral infection, antibiotics do not work).

What is the role of children in the transmission of SARS-CoV-2?

It has been found that children commonly transmit the infection to other children and the elderly. This is applicable to all respiratory infections such as influenza and also true for SARS-CoV-2. The studies have found that the risk of transmission in pairs of the same age and gender is higher. Part of this could be explained by the fact that people of the same age intermix more frequently.

As and when school reopens, what specific preventive measures need to be taken?

In addition to all standard CABs, special efforts should be made to educate both students and schoolteachers on public health and social measures in preventing the transmission. Specifically, schoolchildren and college-going youth should reach out to adult family members and faculty members in order to clarify their fears and concerns related to COVID-19.

What are the broader principles on ventilation and air conditioning to prevent COVID-19?

A regular maintenance service of the heating, ventilation and air conditioning should be done. The indoor setting of these systems should be altered to reduce the recirculation of air. In general there should be good cross-ventilation and, in case of central air conditioning, good air exchange with fresh air.

Can the virus that causes COVID-19 be transmitted through the air?

Studies suggest that the virus that causes COVID-19 is mainly transmitted through contact with respiratory droplets, rather than through the air.

How long can the virus survive on surfaces?

Studies have shown that the COVID-19 virus can survive for up to seventy-two hours on plastic and stainless steel, less than four hours on copper and less than twenty-four hours on cardboard. However, this may vary under different conditions (for instance, the type of surface, temperature or humidity of the environment). It is important to understand that some of these studies have been conducted in ideal laboratory conditions, which are very different from real-life situations. It is important to clean and sanitize commonly touched surfaces.

What is the difference between physical distancing, self-quarantine and self-isolation?

Physical distancing means maintaining a distance in crowded settings. Quarantine means restricting activities or separating people who are not ill themselves but may have been exposed to COVID-19. Isolation refers to separating people who are ill with symptoms of COVID-19 and may be infectious.

How effective are thermal scanners in detecting people infected with COVID-19?

Thermal scanners do not detect whether a person has COVID-19 or not. These scanners measure the body temperature and identify those who have fever (that is, have a higher than normal body temperature). Fever is one of the symptoms of COVID-19 and could be due to many other reasons. Thermal scanners cannot identify a COVID-19-infected person who does not have fever. It may take between two and fourteen days (although, it is usually between five to eight days) for people who are infected to become sick and develop fever. A proportion of them may never do so. Only an identified test can confirm COVID-19.

Can COVID-19 be transmitted in a swimming pool?

The coronavirus is a droplet infection which needs to be inhaled to cause the disease. It is believed that chlorination of water can kill the virus. Yet, there are many unknowns and our knowledge is continuously evolving.

Is there any special protocol to follow for washing fruits and vegetables?

Wash them thoroughly as you would do otherwise, with clean water. Do not use detergent or other harmful materials on fruits and vegetables. Wash your hands properly after washing fruits and vegetables and avoid touching your face while washing fruits and vegetables.

Box 11.6 Busting Myths: A Few Facts about COVID-19

- There is no evidence that exposure to the sun or temperatures higher than 35°C offers protection from COVID-19. If one tries to do so, it can cause sunburn and heatstroke.

- Almost 98–99 per cent of people with COVID-19 recover. However, a small proportion may develop long-term complications, termed long COVID.

- Hand dryers are not known to be effective in killing the SARS-CoV-2 virus. Similarly, ultraviolet (UV) lamps do not disinfect hands or other areas of your skin. These are not a replacement for handwashing with soap and water or disinfecting with sanitizers for 20 to 40 seconds. Rather, UV radiation can cause skin irritation and damage your eyes.

Can COVID-19 spread from food? How safe is food ordered from outside?

There is currently no confirmed case of COVID-19 transmitted through food or food packaging. Packaged food and food items are unlikely to transmit the virus. There is no evidence to suggest that COVID-19 is transmitted through food and water. However, considering that the containers we use may hold and transmit the virus to others, it is essential that we remain cautious. Anyone with suspected symptoms like cough and cold should avoid cooking food for others. One should properly clean the surface of the packaged food as a precaution.

Is it safe to receive a courier package?

Yes. Evidence says that the likelihood of an infected person contaminating commercial goods is low. The risk of catching COVID-19 from a package that has moved through, travelled and been exposed to different conditions and temperatures is low. The outer surface of the package should be properly cleaned.

Can COVID-19 spread from shoes?

Evidence available till now indicates that the likelihood of COVID-19 being spread through shoes and then infecting others is low. As a precautionary measure, families with infants and young children should store shoes where children cannot reach them.

Can I catch COVID-19 from my pet?

It is a disease transmitted from human-to-human through droplet infection as well as through surface contact. Though there have been a few cases of transmission reported from domestic animals to humans, the details on additional factors are not available for those settings. Studies have found that cats and dogs can get the virus from human beings. Researchers have cautioned against the over-interpretation of these findings. As of now, limited evidence suggests that animals do not contribute to wider spread of infection.

Can COVID-19 be transmitted by houseflies and mosquitoes?

There is no evidence that COVID-19 can be transmitted through houseflies and mosquitoes.

Does the virus spread through air travel?

There are reported cases of transfer of the virus through air travel. However, emerging evidence indicates that the risk is lower than thought earlier. In fact, as a rule, the chances of infection increase with an increase in touchpoints. It is important to follow all the preventive measures.

How many times in a day should I wash my hands?

There is no rule as such. Wash or sanitize the hands on a regular basis.

Should one shower after returning from every public place, mall or a hospital?

It is not necessary to shower every time after returning from public places. However, this should be looked at on a case-to-case basis and the risk one poses to family members. If there are high-risk members, it may help to change clothes and take a shower. Every visit to the hospital does not mandate a shower on return but it can be done as a precautionary measure. However, healthcare workers who spend long hours in hospital and potential cases may consider changing clothes and taking a shower on return.

Are there special home remedies and food items which can prevent and cure COVID-19?

There is no food item known or scientifically proven to prevent or cure COVID-19. Many concoctions have been recommended at various forums, mostly as preventive measures. While these could provide nutrition, and be beneficial for a balanced diet, they are not yet scientifically proven to prevent and treat COVID-19.

How relevant is the discussion on a country or city reaching peak cases?

It is difficult to say whether a country or city has reached peak cases. From an individual's perspective, it is not very relevant as one has to follow precautions irrespective of the peak. There is near consensus among experts that for a country the size of

India, a single peak is unlikely. Different cities or states may experience peak at different times. Our understanding of the virus is evolving. The reduction in death rates can be attributed to improved health services, more testing and early detection of cases. It is a good sign but not linked to the peak of cases.

There is a lot of discussion on 'social vaccine' against COVID-19. What is that?

Vaccine is a pharmacological preventive measure to protect from a disease. Non-pharmacological preventive measures like handwashing, face masks and physical distancing in the context of COVID-19 have been at times described as 'social vaccines'. These social and personal measures are as important as a vaccine in stopping the spread of the infection.

Is the COVID-19 in India different from the rest of the world?

If we go by genome analysis, three major strains of CoV-2 are circulating in India. These strains are linked to the virus that originated in Wuhan, Italy and Iran. However, there is no reason to believe that the disease in India is any different from that in any other part of the world. Though minor changes in genes are part of the virus's evolution process.

What can be learnt from the second wave of COVID-19 in Europe and some other countries in late October 2020?

By the end of October 2020, there was a fresh wave of cases in many countries in Europe and the third wave in USA.

Many of these countries are reporting far higher number of cases than the first wave in March–April 2020. Thereafter, the cases had declined for some time. In the months following the first peak, the countries had started routine activities including inter-country travel (though within Europe), travelling, large gatherings within countries, and nearly all activities were open including bars and restaurants. There were also reports of reduced adherence to public health and social measures. With fresh and even bigger peaks in many countries, the national governments have once again put restrictions and lockdowns. The activities have been curtailed.

In the last few months, what has been learnt is that the virus follows a particular cycle and it takes a few weeks before the number rises sufficiently to cause widespread infection. The message is that until the pandemic is fully over, we need to follow recommended non-pharmacological interventions (face masks, handwashing and physical distancing) to protect ourselves and our family members as well as to prevent another peak in our city, state and country. Countries that have strictly adhered to these measures like Taiwan and Vietnam have not seen a spike in cases as reported in Europe.

How long will the pandemic last? For how long do we have to follow precautions?

It is difficult to predict as this is a completely novel virus. The Spanish Flu in 1918–19 lasted nearly eighteen months and had around three waves. SARS-CoV-2 is different, and we hope that once a vaccine is developed and most people in the world are vaccinated, the pandemic would be over. It is understandable that people are getting impatient. Following CABs can be irksome. However, as long as the virus is causing the pandemic, we cannot afford to relax. Any relaxation in norms of physical distancing, wearing of face masks and handwashing could lead to a spike in the virus and undo all the good work done so far.

Disclaimer

The information used in the main text of the chapters and for the Frequently Asked Questions, as and where possible, has been cited. The authors have made an attempt to cite the most updated and reliable sources including peer-reviewed medical journals. A lot of information on the aspects covered in this chapter and the book have been made available on the official websites of the Union ministry of health and family welfare, Government of India, and those of the World Health Organization (WHO) and the United States Centers for Disease Control and Prevention (US CDC). We have also sourced some information from these websites and acknowledge them with thanks.

Afterword

The Future of Healthcare and Humanity Is Interlinked

Having lived through the COVID-19 pandemic for so many months, we all wish things to return to 'normal' as early as possible. However, one can ask a slightly philosophical question: what is normal? A world without the Internet was normal, except for a select few, in the 1980s. A world without widespread mobile telephone use was normal twenty years ago. HIV/AIDS changed our practice of how blood banks functioned and what practices we follow with regard to sex. Having experienced SARS-CoV-2, our thinking and our daily routines have changed.

When we compare the present and the probable future with pre-COVID-19 times, we have a window of opportunities at all levels—as individuals, as a society and as a nation—for three things: reject, revive and innovate.

- **Reject.** There are activities and actions that need to be rejected or reduced as we look forward to a new normal. Recognizing our global connectivity, we need to think about activities that led to where we are and see what we can do to change that. Our environment matters, climate change is real—deforestation and rampant and unplanned urbanization are future disasters in waiting. What can we do to change and advocate for change?

  We can and must reject the drivers of lifestyle diseases—fast food, lack of exercise, stress and ignoring mental health. Promoting health and reducing drivers of ill health is the best way to ensure that risks of severe disease are reduced.

- **Revive.** There are things which need to continue as before, such as economic and social activities. The revival of the economy in a sustainable way has to be underpinned by an improvement in the conditions of living of the most impoverished, instead of further enriching the already rich. Investments in health and education transform economies, and while this does not happen in election cycles, it is essential that scientists, economists, health workers and the public make this the keystone of our collective future.

- **Innovate.** The future needs new tools and new behaviours, whether it is better health surveillance or raising the consistency of handwashing, we need to find solutions that make their adoption easy at all levels from governments to individuals.

In India, in particular, the attempt to transform the health system is embodied in continuing the initiatives started under the National Health Mission, supplemented by additional measures under the Ayushman Bharat programme. Primary healthcare and public health services need to be strengthened in an accelerated manner under the HWCs of the Ayushman Bharat programme. The health initiatives need further strengthening and linking, not just across all healthcare providers in India, but with other sectors including education, women and child development, and industry. An isolated approach that views development as being driven by the government alone ignores huge resources and strengths that exist beyond the government.

There is evidence aplenty that epidemics and pandemics impact the poor, the marginalized, women and children the most. Building for their protection requires a reimagining of the base of the Indian health system—one that is equitable, affordable and accessible. This may sound like a pipe dream, but there are examples of nations achieving better health parameters with limited resources.

Health is not found in hospitals, it is built at home. Water supply, sanitation, protection from pollution, screening services and mental health support are all essential for a healthy mind and body that can handle the challenges of ill health when it occurs. In addition to the provision of healthcare, the government needs to facilitate nutrition, a better built environment, and better training of the workforce. These are areas where good policies and effective implementation are as important as direct investments.

In the provision of services, public health requires interconnected systems that share quality data based on which decisions can be made or actions taken. At the moment, fragmentation and vertical programmes lead to duplication of resources and efforts. It is time for a rethink to develop more efficient approaches that will provide the connected, resilient systems that we need to control disease and promote health, for everyone and everywhere.

In September 2020, the journal *Science* published the findings of a US study on the effect of reduced motor vehicular traffic on birds singing.[1] The authors reported that due to shutdowns and other actions taken to control the pandemic, the noise level in a city had dramatically reduced to the level observed in the mid-1950s. This had resulted in the birds singing at lower amplitudes and still being heard by people far away. The authors concluded that 'behavioural traits can change rapidly in response to newly favourable conditions'.

We have written this book to communicate a similar message. If the birds can change their behaviour so quickly, we humans should do better in recognizing the signals given by nature. The COVID-19 pandemic indicates the damage we have done to our planet and to ourselves. It is our responsibility to continue to learn and develop ways of improving our world, our health systems and our health.

Much has changed; we are in a difficult time. But there is no need to panic. Instead, there are many reasons to hope that science and technology will provide the solutions we need. Together we can create a better and healthier world for everyone.

---

[1]   E.P. Derryberry, et al., *Science*, 2020. Available at https://science. sciencemag.org/content/early/2020/09/23/science.abd5777.